"Digital health is revitalizing the increasingly demanding patient. How the system and professionals face the challenge of humanizing healthcare is a major question, to which this book seeks a transformative answer. It is a highly recommended introduction to the paradigm shift."

Jordi Farré Coma, *Universitat Rovira i Virgili, Spain*

"This book offers brilliant analyses of the ways in which digitalization changes all healthcare communication and how the digitalization of healthcare communication alters the sociocultural understanding of patienthood. It provides anyone interested in healthcare communication with relevant information and new directions of study."

Valentina Marinescu, *University of Bucharest, Romania*

"This book departs from the traditional perspective of health communication dominated by an industrial view presenting the patient as a passive recipient of assistance from above. Focusing on patienthood, the authors reverse the perspective to a patient-centred approach facilitated by digital opportunities."

Kaarle Nordenstreng, *Tampere University, Finland*

Healthcare and Patient Communication in the Digital Era

This book provides a social and cultural theoretical framework for the digitalization of healthcare communication from a patient-centred perspective.

Through empirical case studies, the book outlines the experiences of patients as the digitalization of healthcare communication re-spatializes and re-temporalizes care and reconstructs patienthood and ill health. To demonstrate how changes in communication impact health and illness, the book examines the digitalization process from three viewpoints. Firstly, it illustrates how the digitalization of illness enhances the availability of information and peer support, which increases patient empowerment. Secondly, it shows how the digitalization of disease transforms signs of disease in a patient's body into electronic data, increases the distance between the disease and the patient, and enables diagnosis without a healthcare professional touching a patient's body. Finally, it explains how the digitalization of sickness changes the power relations founded in health and reconfigures health citizenship.

Filling a theoretical gap in health communication scholarship, this book will be of interest to academics and postgraduate students in the fields of Health Communication, Digital Communication, Communication Studies, and Health Sciences. The book also offers healthcare professionals new perspectives to respond to the increasing communicative duties arising from the digitalization of healthcare communication.

Sinikka Torkkola is a Senior Research Fellow in the Faculty of Information Technology and Communication Sciences at Tampere University, Finland. She is also an Adjunct Professor in the Faculty of Humanities at the University of Oulu, Finland.

Anna Sendra Toset is a Project Manager in the Faculty of Information Technology and Communication Sciences at Tampere University, Finland.

Routledge Research in Health Communication

1 **Communicating Women's Health**
Social and Cultural Norms that Influence Health Decisions
Edited by Annette Madlock Gatison

2 **Culture, Migration, and Health Communication in a Global Context**
Edited by Yuping Mao and Rukhsana Ahmed

3 **Immigration and Strategic Public Health Communication**
Lessons from the Transnational Seguro Popular Project
Edited by Robert C. Smith, Don J. Waisanen, and Guillermo Yrizar Barbosa

4 **Post-AIDS Discourse in Health Communication**
Sociocultural Interpretations
Edited by Ambar Basu, Andrew R. Spieldenner and Patrick J. Dillon

5 **Global Health Communication for Immigrants and Refugees**
Cases, Theories, and Strategies
Edited by Do Kyun David Kim and Gary L. Kreps

6 **Humor and Health in the Media**
Raising the Question, Should Illness be Funny?
Malynnda A. Johnson

7 **Covid-19 Misinformation Flows**
Challenges and Options for Reconstructing and Disseminating Mediated Messages
Emmanuel K. Ngwainmbi

8 **Healthcare and Patient Communication in the Digital Era**
A Patienthood and Patient Perspective
Sinikka Torkkola and Anna Sendra Toset

Healthcare and Patient Communication in the Digital Era

A Patienthood and Patient Perspective

Sinikka Torkkola and Anna Sendra Toset

Routledge
Taylor & Francis Group
NEW YORK AND LONDON

First published 2026
by Routledge
605 Third Avenue, New York, NY 10158

and by Routledge
4 Park Square, Milton Park, Abingdon, Oxon, OX14 4RN

Routledge is an imprint of the Taylor & Francis Group, an informa business

Data availability statement:
Data sharing is not applicable to this book as no new data were created or analysed in this study.

ISBN: 978-1-032-85733-6 (hbk)
ISBN: 978-1-032-85734-3 (pbk)
ISBN: 978-1-003-51960-7 (ebk)

DOI: 10.4324/9781003519607

Typeset in Times New Roman
by Apex CoVantage, LLC

Contents

Preface ix

1 **Introduction** 1

1.1 Patient, client, citizen? 2
1.2 Differences between "digitization" and "digitalization" 5
1.3 Digitalization of healthcare communication 6
1.4 The future of healthcare 8
1.5 Structure of the book 9

2 **Communication and ill health** 18

2.1 Communicating ill health 22
2.2 Communicating health and illness 24
2.3 Construction of patienthood in digital healthcare communication 30

3 **Digitalization of illness: from paternalism to empowerment** 37

3.1 The experience of being ill from the perspective of the patient 38
3.2 Narratives to construct and make sense of the experience of being ill 40
3.3 Digitalizing the experience of being ill 42
3.4 Risks associated with the digitalization of illness 46
3.5 The consolidation of participatory patienthood 49

4 From the medical gaze to the digital gaze 57

4.1 The birth of modern medicine 58
4.2 Digitalization of medical information delivery 60
4.3 Digitalization of medical care 64
4.4 Towards joint expertise 69

5 Digitalization of sickness: renegotiating health citizenship 79

5.1 The experience of being ill from the perspective of society 81
5.2 Understanding health citizenship 83
5.3 From health citizenship to digital health citizenship 85
5.4 Beyond the relationship between empowerment and self-discipline 89
5.5 Towards a balanced digital health citizenship 91

6 Patienthood and healthcare communication in the digital era 99

6.1 Digitalization of communicative tasks 102
6.2 Digitalization of patienthood 105

Index *110*

Preface

This book is the result of almost ten years of collaboration that started when Anna emailed Sinikka in September 2016 with a proposal for a research stay at the University of Tampere (Tampere, Finland), now known as Tampere University since 2019. At that time, Anna was doing her PhD on health communication and social media at the Universitat Rovira i Virgili (Tarragona, Spain), and Sinikka had just completed a four-year project on the same topic at the University of Tampere. Almost one year later, Sinikka and Anna met in person for the first time in August 2017 during the NordMedia conference, which happened to be organized at the University of Tampere. The rest is history.

Healthcare and Patient Communication in the Digital Era provides an overview of how digitalization changes all healthcare communication between care receivers, care providers, and the institution, and it reveals in what ways these temporal and spatial reorientations in healthcare communication alter the sociocultural understanding of patienthood. Given that the patient is at the core of healthcare communication, the perspective of the patient is essential for understanding the intricacies of healthcare communication. This book not only offers an analysis of the digitalization of healthcare communication from the patient's viewpoint but also answers the demand for more theoretical work in the field of health communication and discusses the generous empirical research available on communication and the digitalization of healthcare.

Since September 2016, Sinikka and Anna have worked together on numerous occasions, including publishing as co-authors on a recurrent basis; jointly guest editing a special issue on communication and digital health for the *Catalan Journal of Communication & Cultural Studies* with a colleague from South Africa; collaborating in a project that looked at the significance of non-knowing and ignorance for professional work; jointly establishing the first-ever temporary working group on health communication for NordMedia 2019 with colleagues from Denmark, Norway, and Sweden; co-chairing together a health communication working group at Mevi-päivät 2024; and disseminating the results of their research at multiple conferences (e.g., IAMCR, ECREA). Moreover, both Sinikka and Anna have acted as abstract reviewers for the Health Communication Working Group of the IAMCR conference on numerous occasions. Sinikka also acted as vice chair of the aforementioned working group between 2019 and 2023.

For Sinikka, health communication was not her first interest; it was journalism, on which she wrote her master's thesis. When she graduated just after the economic crisis of the 1990s, there were no full-time jobs for journalists, so she combined a part-time researcher job at the Department of Public Health with working as a freelance journalist for one television show on health, a role she gained in part due to her background as a registered nurse. Around that time, the Research and Development unit of the University of Tampere launched a competition for research ideas, so Sinikka entered with an idea concerning critical health journalism. She won the competition and was subsequently hired for two months to complete a research plan for the PhD based on the submitted idea. Back then, there were barely any health communication scholars in Finland, and the situation nowadays remains similar. However, Sinikka started a cooperation on health communication together with a couple of colleagues, organized conference sessions for the Finnish Conference of Media and Communication Research (Mevi-päivät) and co-edited with Leena Mikkola a special issue for the leading Finnish journal on communication and media studies, *Tiedotustutkimus* (now known as *Media & viestintä*). She also edited the first Finnish book on health communication in 2002 – titled *Terveysviestintä* – and co-authored the first and only Finnish guidebook for writers of patient leaflets, also published in 2002. Since completing her 2008 doctoral dissertation on hospital newspapers and the theory of health journalism, Sinikka has mostly done research on health communication, especially from the viewpoint of digitalization and social media. Health communication theory (or rather, the lack of it) has inspired Sinikka since the start of her career. The ideas on the relation between communication and ill health present in this book were already born during the writing process of the monograph for her doctoral dissertation.

For Anna, her interest in health communication was ignited on the day she began to work as a research assistant for the research group ALGOS at the Universitat Rovira i Virgili. The research group, interested in the study and treatment of paediatric pain, inspired Anna to find the theme of her dissertation. Her father being diagnosed with a rare disease contributed to her choice of topic too. The idea that patients were using social media to manage their illnesses became the cornerstone of her research interests, which focus on studying digitalization processes from different perspectives (media and communication studies, philosophy, and information studies), especially in the context of healthcare. When she started her PhD, Anna was in a similar situation as Sinikka, as back then there were barely any health communication scholars in Spain. However, and especially thanks to the tireless work of Dr Daniel Catalán Matamoros, Anna was able to attend several conferences on health communication organized at the national level during her PhD. At one of these conferences (I Jornadas Nacionales de Comunicación en Salud, organized in 2016), Anna won an award for the best oral communication presented at the event for her presentation of a study that analysed how healthcare organizations communicate pain-related messages on social media. After her doctoral dissertation, she also organized in 2019 a national symposium on health communication – titled Communication and health: Innovative experiences – at the Universitat Rovira i Virgili together with her PhD supervisor. Moreover, Anna has been a member of the editorial committee for the Spanish journal on health communication *Revista Española de Comunicación en Salud* since 2019.

In view of this, it could be said that this book has been in the making over the last two decades. The process of writing *Healthcare and Patient Communication in the Digital Era* is not only a result of the multiple in-person and virtual meetings, shared online documents, and an undetermined number of readings since the first encounter with their editor, but also a result of all the activities that Sinikka and Anna have carried out throughout the years driven by their common interest in health communication. During this time, many people have also engaged with Sinikka's and Anna's research. This book would certainly not have been possible without their inspiration and support.

The first person Sinikka and Anna would like to thank is Dr Anna-Maria Mäki-Kuutti. While Sinikka and Anna are listed as the only authors of this book, the writing of *Healthcare and Patient Communication in the Digital Era* would never have happened without the help of Dr Mäki-Kuutti, with whom Sinikka and Anna wrote a presentation for the IAMCR 2023 conference in Lyon. This presentation was the seed that gave rise to the creation of the book presented here. Unfortunately, because of other duties, Dr Mäki-Kuutti could not continue in the project. Her work on health and gender and health and society particularly inspired Sinikka and Anna during the writing process of this book.

Sinikka and Anna would also like to extend their special thanks to Dr Jaana Parviainen and Dr Jordi Farré Coma for the discussions around the topic of this book. In particular, Dr Parviainen's expertise in philosophy and Dr Farré Coma's expertise in risk communication helped broaden the scope of their work. A special memory for Anna is from December 2022, when she spent more than two hours with Sinikka and Jordi talking about the digitalization of healthcare communication in one of the offices of the Universitat Rovira i Virgili, her academic home.

Furthermore, Sinikka and Anna would like to thank their international colleagues for engaging in meaningful discussions on health communication over the years, especially Dr Eliza Govender for co-editing the special issue on communication and digital health previously described, Dr Robert W. Vaagan for arranging a two-day research workshop at Oslo Metropolitan University in 2019 to talk about the digitalization of healthcare communication, and Dr Alessandro Lovari for participating in rich conversations on social media and health communication that started in Lugano during the ECREA 2018 conference and culminated in the publication of an article along with Jordi and Robert.

Likewise, Sinikka would like to thank Dr Valentina Marinescu and Dr Ramona Marinache, with whom she had fruitful discussions on health communication during Sinikka's research visit at the University of Bucharest in the autumn of 2019. Sinikka would also like to extend her thanks to Dr Yolanda Paul and Dr SubbaRao M Gavaravarapu, with whom she collaborated in the Health Communication Working Group of the IAMCR conference alongside Dr Eliza Govender.

For her part, Anna would like to express her deepest gratitude to her supervisors since the start of her research career, especially for their endless support. In addition to Jaana and Jordi, Anna's supervisors have also included Dr Sanna Kumpulainen and Dr Sylvie Grosjean. All their invaluable insights, sustained encouragement, and crucial advice both during and beyond Anna's PhD have not only continued to inspire Anna in her academic life, but they have also helped her to become the researcher she is today.

In addition, Sinikka and Anna would like to thank Tampere University, especially the Faculty of Information Technology and Communication Sciences, as well as Dr Iiris Ruoho and Dr Marko Ala-Fossi (former and current head of the Communication Sciences unit), for giving them the time and space to write this book.

Lastly, Sinikka and Anna would like to thank the Locum Bildarkiv (Locum Image Archive) for providing the photograph of the Huddinge Hospital (© 1971) featured in Chapter 1 as well as the newspaper *Aamulehti* for providing the photograph of one of the operating rooms of the Coxa Hospital for Joint Replacement (© 2023) featured in Chapter 4. They also wish to thank their proofreader, Matthew James, for carefully reviewing the chapters; their editor at Routledge, Alexandra de Brauw, who made this book possible; and their editorial assistant, Zoya Gayle, for her guidance during the preparation of this publication.

Sinikka would like to end this preface by thanking her spouse, Jussi, and their 20-year-old cat, Vili, who make home a place to love and to be loved. For her part, Anna would like to end this preface by expressing her enormous gratitude to her parents, Carme and Àngel, and to her partner, Dilara, for their continued love, help, and support.

Sinikka Torkkola and Anna Sendra Toset
Tampere, Finland
May 2025

1 Introduction

> An airport works like a chain of logical functions, with the passengers arriving, checking in, going through passport control, buying duty-free alcohol, taking an export beer in the bar, relieving themselves, then standing at the gate to choose a seat on the plane, preferably near to emergency exit.
>
> Is there a similar chain of logical function in a hospital? Probably. A hospital is constructed like a sorting office, the person arriving first having to produce a ticket to say he or she is ill. What is meant by being ill? What is disease? What does a disease look like? This is where definitions part company. But after what is sometimes a rather lengthy process at the check-in desk, someone in the hospital, usually a doctor, decides whether the illness exists or not. The person who is not ill is consequently well and has to go back home.
>
> (Jersild, 1987, p. 8)

In the novel *House of Babel*, the hospital (see Figure 1.1) is compared to the airport and the patient to a travelling passenger. A patient whose illness is a ticket to the hospital is transported like a package through the gigantic hospital without adequate communication with the doctors and nurses. The novel, published in Swedish in 1978, opened a keen discussion concerning the hospital and the dehumanization of the patient in Sweden and the other Nordic countries (Autio, 1980; Jersild, 1982; Sevilä, 1980).

After the publication of the novel, the author, P. C. Jersild, also a physician specialized in psychiatry, went on a discussion tour about the topics of the novel all over Sweden and met thousands of Swedish citizens criticizing both hospitals and healthcare more generally (Jersild, 1982). Today, the novel still inspires discussion around modern hospitals, patienthood, and medical technology (Bosseldal, 2006; Dussauge, 2004; Svensson, 2024). The critique inspired by the novel concerns not only the hospital as a bureaucratic organization or a medical technology but also the communication within the hospital and between the doctors, nurses, and patients, in which the patient is invited mostly to perform as a passive, voiceless carrier of disease.

DOI: 10.4324/9781003519607-1

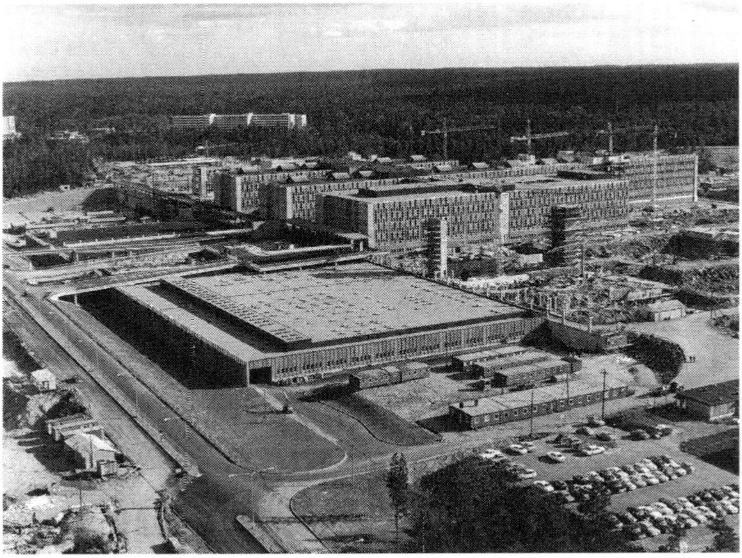

Figure 1.1 The Swedish hospital Huddinge, located in Stockholm, was the exemplar for P. C. Jersild's novel *House of Babel*. In the 1960s, the hospital was the largest construction project in Scandinavia. From "Huddinge sjukhus – lika stort som Gamla stan [Huddinge Hospital – as big as the Old Town]", by G. Nordin (photo) & M. Ljungström (text), January 25, 2021, *Locum* (https://www.locum.se/om-oss/press/nyheter/2021/huddinge-sjukhus-historia/). Photograph by the Locum Bildarkiv (© 1971). Reprinted with permission.

The interaction between a care provider/doctor/nurse and a care receiver/patient/client is at the core of healthcare communication (Fleischer et al., 2009; Ha & Longnecker, 2010). The COVID-19 pandemic showed the complexity of the communication environment of healthcare communication (see Figure 1.2) and forced organizations to modify their communicative actions and information delivery processes to be more transparent, as required by citizens, media, companies, and other authorities (Aguerrebere et al., 2024).

1.1 Patient, client, citizen?

The term "patient", as we understand it today, got its meaning during the foundation of modern medicine, as Michel Foucault (1963/1994) described in *The Birth of the Clinic*. Etymologically, "patient" means a sufferer (Sontag, 2002, p. 123). The word "patient" comes from the Latin *patiens*, from the present participle of *pati* (i.e., to suffer), perhaps akin to the Greek *pēma* (Merriam-Webster, n.d.). In 1350, the word "patient" meant "enduring pain,

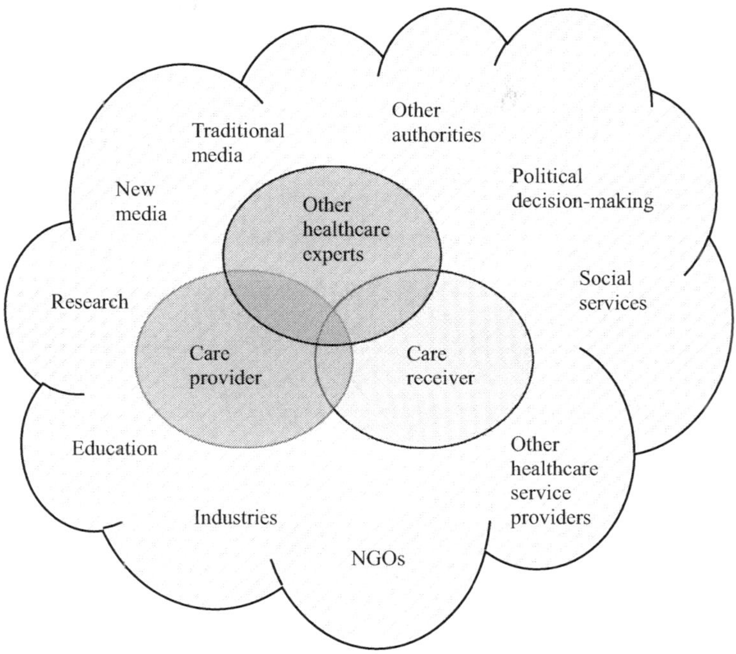

Figure 1.2 The communication environment of healthcare communication. Created by the authors.

affliction, inconvenience, etc., calmly, without discontent or complaint; characterized by or showing such endurance" (Oxford English Dictionary, n.d.). With the advance of modern medicine, the patient as a suffering subject was put aside, and the patient as a carrier of disease under the medical gaze entered the scene (Foucault, 1963/1994). As Sharf and Street Jr (1997, p. 4) have pointed out, the patient connotes a passive or helpless object who compliantly receives medical directives.

Since the 1980s, there has been an ongoing discussion regarding a more active and co-equal role for patients (Sharf & Street Jr, 1997). Nowadays, there seems to be a consensus for a more active form of patienthood (Sosnowy, 2014), but there is no consensus on which word would be the most suitable for a subject promoting health, using healthcare services or receiving medical treatment or care of another kind (Costa et al., 2019; Flores-Sandoval et al., 2021; Hogg, 1999; Sharf & Street Jr, 1997). Christine Hogg (1999, p. 2) has pointed out that there is no word that everyone may comfortably use to describe the individual receiver of healthcare. "Patient", "client", "customer", "consumer", and "user" are all used, and each has different implications. "Patient" implies passivity and an unequal power relationship between the care provider and care receiver (Hogg, 1999). Sharf and Street Jr (1997) compare the terms "patient", "client", "healthcare customer", "citizen", and "partner", each of them carrying a different kind of burden, but end up using the word "patient".

Today, the term "care receiver" seems to have replaced those other terms at least in health communication writings. Despite that, and depending on the context, in this book we use as synonyms the terms "patient", "care receiver", "citizen", and "customer". From the viewpoint of medicine, a person using healthcare services is a patient. An activist from a patient organization can be a patient, too. A person shopping at the market is naturally a customer, and an individual participating in the public discussion at the general level is a citizen. Moreover, a care receiver is an individual interacting with physicians, nurses, and other healthcare professionals.

A similar discussion has been held on the word "health" (Sendra, 2019). The use of this term to describe the experience of being well (see, for instance, the definition provided by the WHO in 1948)[1] implies a "complete" absence of illness. Thus, according to this and other definitions, the state of being a patient falls outside the use of this term (Smith, 2008). Moreover, in a world where "[a]geing with chronic illnesses has become the norm" (Huber et al., 2011, Limitations of WHO definition section, para. 3), healthcare communication is also affected by the term "health". As a citizen, a care receiver is continuously exposed to information (e.g., both through traditional and new media) on how to achieve this "complete" absence of illness. As a patient, the care receiver is encouraged to use healthcare services to return to this "complete" absence of illness. As a client, the care receiver is increasingly offered data (e.g., a menu including the number of calories a meal has) to assess how to maintain this "complete" absence of illness. While the use of this term to describe the experience of being well has been previously criticized by care providers (e.g., Huber et al., 2011), the word "health" remains unadjusted. However, a more recent study defined "health" as "[a] structural, functional and emotional state that is compatible with effective life as an individual and as a member of society" (McCartney et al., 2019, p. 24). In this new explanation, the "complete" absence of illness is no longer required.

In this regard, it should also be noted that there are different types of health. On the one hand, there is human health, which corresponds to the definitions of health provided by the WHO (1948) and McCartney et al. (2019). On the other hand, there is environmental health, which corresponds to "the field of public health that addresses physical, chemical, biological, social, and psychosocial factors in the environment" (Frumkin, 2016, p. 58). Likewise, there is animal health, which corresponds to the maintenance of animal welfare and the prevention of animal diseases (EFSA, 2024). Human, environmental, and animal health converge in what the WHO defines as the One Health approach, where "the health of humans, domestic and wild animals, plants, and the wider environment (including ecosystems) are closely linked and interdependent" (WHO, n.d.). Although the term "One Health" was officially coined in 2008 (CDC, 2024), its relevance became particularly emphasized during the COVID-19 pandemic (Lefrançois et al., 2023; Ohia & Uwalaka, 2021). In relation to this approach, some authors have also started to engage in a more-than-human perspective to analyse ill health (Lupton, 2022a), arguing for the development of a digital One Health (Lupton, 2022b). In this book, we will focus on exploring the digitalization of healthcare communication in the context of human health.

1.2 Differences between "digitization" and "digitalization"

Although "digitization" and "digitalization" are closely related terms, Brennen and Kreiss (2016) argue for a distinct definition of these concepts. For these authors, digitization is used to "refer to the technical process of converting streams of analog information into digital bits of 1s and 0s with discrete and discontinuous values" (Brennen & Kreiss, 2016, Digitization section, para. 1). Conversely, digitalization is used to "refer to the structuring of many and diverse domains of social life around digital communication and media infrastructures" (Brennen & Kreiss, 2016, Digitalization section, para. 1). Against this background, one could argue that digitization is a process that has been present at least since the 1930s, when the first modern computers were invented (Britannica, 2025). The physicist and mathematician John Vincent Atanasoff is credited with inventing the first electronic computer in 1939 (Britannica, 2025). However, digitalization is a rather more recent phenomenon that is specifically concerned "with the ways that digital media variously structure, shape, and influence the contemporary world" (Brennen & Kreiss, 2016, Digitalization section, para. 1). Therefore, in this book, we focus on digitalization instead of digitization, as we are interested in discussing how digital media "structure, shape, and influence" healthcare communication.

In the context of healthcare digitalization, there are different ways "in which digital and mobile technologies are being used to support health" (WHO, 2023, p. 1), both at the individual and organizational levels. According to the classification of *Digital Interventions, Services, and Applications in Health* made by the WHO (2023), healthcare digitalization is organized around three axes: health system challenges (which represent the gaps affecting the efficiency of the organization and delivery of healthcare, such as availability), digital health interventions (which represent the capabilities of digital health for supporting the organization and delivery of healthcare), and service and application types (which represent the architecture of digital health, such as registries and directories). For the digital health interventions axis, the WHO (2023) further organizes these capabilities according to their primary end-user, including persons (i.e., care receivers), healthcare providers (i.e., care providers), health management and support personnel, and data services. While this classification proves useful for educating and training primary end-users on digital health as well as supporting the implementation of digital health interventions in the organization and delivery of healthcare, the maturity of healthcare digitalization remains to be measured (Maaß et al., 2024). Assessing the maturity of healthcare digitalization is crucial, as it can "empower decision-makers to make informed choices, optimize resource allocation, and drive innovation in healthcare delivery" (Maaß et al., 2024, Abstract section).

However, despite the focus of our book, we acknowledge that contemporary healthcare communication is influenced by the processes of both digitization and digitalization. One example is electronic health records. The deployment of electronic health records is an example of digitization, while the use of electronic health records for the provision of healthcare services is an example of digitalization. From the perspective of digitalization, electronic health records not only improve healthcare communication between care providers (e.g., in cases of multi-speciality care) but also between care providers and care receivers (Gavrilov et al., 2020). In other words, electronic health records "structure" healthcare communication. Another example is electronic consultations. The deployment of electronic consultations is an example of digitization, while the use of electronic consultations for the provision of healthcare services is an example of digitalization. From the viewpoint of digitalization, electronic consultations impact the ways healthcare services are usually provided (e.g., face-to-face vs electronic consultation), affecting both the medical practices of care providers (e.g., learning how to diagnose without a body) and the healthcare management practices of care receivers (e.g., learning how to be more autonomous). In other words, electronic consultations both "shape" and "influence" healthcare communication. These are only some of the many examples of the processes of the digitalization of healthcare communication, as we will explore in the next section.

1.3 Digitalization of healthcare communication

As outlined in Figure 1.2, the ongoing digitalization of healthcare communication is changing all levels of communication, not just interactions between care providers and care receivers but also organizational communication. For instance, at the level of interactions between care providers and care receivers, it has previously been observed that telemedicine demands the continuous updating of communication practices and further education for healthcare professionals (Ritunga et al., 2024). Likewise, at the level of organizational communication, data from several studies suggest that the use of social media for public health communication is far from ideal (Fiammenghi et al., 2024; Guidry et al., 2020; Sendra & Farré, 2017), with many healthcare professionals having doubts about how to use these online platforms without compromising their professionalism (Curtis & Gillen, 2019; Torkkola et al., 2024). In this context, telemedicine is only one of the many concepts used to refer to the processes of healthcare digitalization. Other commonly used terms in the literature include "digital health", "eHealth", "Medicine 2.0", "Health 2.0", "telecare", and "m-health" (Iyawa et al., 2016; Lupton, 2013). While these concepts have slightly different meanings (Iyawa et al., 2016), all these terms are related to how digital media "structure, shape, and influence" (Brennen & Kreiss, 2016, Digitalization section, para. 1) healthcare communication.

Other examples of digital technologies altering all levels of communication are digital health platforms, which can exist both at the regional and national levels depending on the healthcare system. Like in the case of e-consultations, a recent study by Alzghaibi (2025) found that perceived barriers to m-health application adoption among care providers include difficult communication with other healthcare professionals and the disruption of the interaction with care receivers. The same study also found that "digital literacy levels significantly influence practitioners' perceptions of these barriers" (Alzghaibi, 2025, Practical Recommendations for Enhancing mHealth Accessibility, Usability, and Integration section, para. 3). Once again, the findings of this and other studies (Curtis & Gillen, 2019; Ritunga et al., 2024; Sendra et al., 2023) highlight the need for the further education of care providers not only in digital (health) literacy but also in media literacy and digital professionalism. As Vaagan et al. (2021, p. 1732) explain, the digitalization of healthcare communication "requires regular training of these individuals [care providers], including the adoption of new digital communication skills". However, care providers are not the only individuals needing further education to cope with the ongoing digitalization of healthcare communication. In the case of care receivers, previous research has shown the importance of health information literacy as "an enabler of acceptance of digital health services" (Eriksson-Backa et al., 2022, p. 322).

In addition to changing all levels of communication, the digitalization of healthcare communication also reorganizes the time and place of healthcare. On the one hand, the digitalization of healthcare communication represents a respatialization of healthcare (Andreassen et al., 2018), where care providers and care receivers are physically separated. This is the case, for example, with e-consultations or virtual wards/hospitals, where a patient can be located anywhere while using healthcare services – at home, in the workplace, or even in public spaces, such as trains or cafés. In other words, with the digitalization of healthcare communication, medical consultations are not only reserved for the clinic. On the other hand, the digitalization of healthcare communication also represents a retemporalization of healthcare, where simultaneous interaction between care providers and care receivers is no longer essential: a patient using a digital health platform or a smart watch can reply to questions from the care provider and gather data produced by the wearable device for diagnosis and treatment at any suitable time. Such respatialization (Andreassen et al., 2018) and retemporalization of healthcare transcend the traditional time and space of healthcare, where Foucault's concept of the clinic "has dispersed to every possible spatial and temporal location" (Lupton, 2013, p. 266).

In this book, we will examine the changes accompanying the digitalization of healthcare communication from the perspective of patients (i.e., illness or communication around the experiences of a condition; see more in Chapter 3), from the perspective of healthcare professionals (i.e., disease or communication around diagnosis and treatment of a condition; see more in Chapter 4), and from the perspective of society (i.e., sickness or communication around the arrangements of healthcare services; see more in Chapter 5). As we will see in the different chapters, these changes have inevitably led to multiple and sometimes conflicting consequences. For example, in a study about smart hospitals, it was found that future developments are seen among the participants both positively for the decentralization of healthcare and negatively for the interaction between care providers and care receivers (Jovy-Klein et al., 2024). Likewise, the digitalization of healthcare communication also risks increasing health inequities (Chidambaram et al., 2024), as this transformation is reconstituting patienthood and ill health at a fundamental level. In this context, Gybel Jensen et al. (2024, Abstract section, para. 5) explain that addressing the digital determinants of health requires one "to be aware of the differences in digital health literacy, focus on simplifying communication with patients and next of kin, and find flexible solutions for citizens who are disadvantaged".

1.4 The future of healthcare

Against this background, what will the future of healthcare look like? By the looks of it, the metaphor of the hospital as an airport and the patient as a travelling passenger described in the novel *House of Babel* might still be relevant when talking about the digitalization of healthcare communication, but it does not represent the future of healthcare – at least not fully. In the future, the hospital will not be an airport but rather a shopping centre where the patient, as a client, will be scanned for the potential presence of ill health, taking current digital technologies such as smart rings and watches one step further. The scanning could be done, for instance, by personalized healthcare companion robots like Baymax, featured in the 2014 animated movie *Big Hero 6* (Hall & Williams, 2014) and later in the 2022 animated series *Baymax!* (Hall, 2022). In both the movie and the series, the robot presents itself to the patient with the following sentence: "Hello! I am Baymax, your personal healthcare companion". Baymax is capable of scanning for symptoms, generating diagnoses, and providing first aid treatment after being alerted to the need for medical attention. Therefore, in the future, the patient will not go to the hospital, but rather, the hospital will come to the patient (respatialization of healthcare).

Furthermore, in the case of needing specialized treatment, homes will be equipped with medical pods, similar in shape to a CT scan, that can be fully operated by the patient like the ones featured in the 2012 Sci-Fi movie *Prometheus* (Scott, 2012), capable of self-diagnosing and performing surgical procedures without human control. In the movie, Dr Elizabeth Shaw (the character played by Noomi Rapace) attempts to use a medical pod to perform a C-section to remove the embryo of an alien from her body. The medical pod also incorporates a procedure for decontamination, thus making the device ready to use again when needed. Consequently, in the future, the patient will not visit the hospital to receive medical and surgical treatment, but rather, the home will become the hospital where the patient will independently use medical equipment (retemporalization of healthcare). As in the case of smart rings and watches, for now, doctors are only capable of performing surgical procedures remotely with the help of a robot (Choi et al., 2018). In this context, *Prometheus* is not the only film or series showing medical pods. Other examples of similar devices include the healing pod featured in the action series *Agents of S.H.I.E.L.D.* (Whedon et al., 2013–2020), albeit in this case, the device is controlled by a semi-robotic being.

1.5 Structure of the book

This book is structured as six chapters: this introduction (the first chapter), four analytical chapters on the digitalization of healthcare communication from general and specific perspectives, and a concluding chapter. Overall, the chapters will examine the digitalization of healthcare communication from the viewpoints of illness, disease, and sickness after presenting how the temporal and spatial reorientations in communication brought by this digital transformation alter the sociocultural understanding of patienthood (i.e., the state of being a patient).

The second chapter, "Communication and ill health", discusses the connections between communication and ill health and analyses the history of the term "health communication" from the origins of the concept in the 1970s up until the present. Inspired by the two perspectives that open an understanding of the term "health communication", we argue that healthcare communication is a sub-field of health communication, including all communicative actions at the interpersonal, organizational, and mass communication levels (e.g., health promotion). This means that the digitalization of healthcare communication is changing the interactions between care receivers, care providers, and (also) institutions, leaving behind the patient–doctor dichotomy through which health and healthcare communication are traditionally understood. Subsequently, the chapter introduces a new theoretical framework of patienthood and health, where expertise, medicalization, and health citizenship are presented as conflicted statuses of ill health in the triad between disease, illness, and sickness. This is done by adopting a culturally oriented understanding of health communication where, guided by the work of Deborah Lutpon (e.g., 1995) and Dutta, M (2008, 2010), health communication is seen as a cultural phenomenon maintaining, producing, and transforming health and illness. The chapter concludes by bringing into focus the perspective of the care receiver, which guides the discussion around the digitalization of healthcare communication for the rest of the book.

The third chapter, "Digitalization of illness: From paternalism to empowerment", explores how the digitalization of healthcare communication has transformed the experience of being ill from the perspective of the patient. Starting with a discussion of what illness means, the chapter then proceeds to illustrate through the case of online communities the five ways in which the digital era is changing the exercise of patienthood by providing opportunities to (1) obtain more informational and emotional social support, (2) co-construct experiential knowledge in a networked manner, (3) address health controversies, (4) talk about illness from non-institutionalized frameworks, and (5) share multimodal expressions of experiential knowledge (Cao & Wang, 2024; Gonzalez-Polledo, 2016; Gonzalez-Polledo & Tarr, 2016; Jackson, 2023; Ressler et al., 2012; Sendra & Farré, 2020; Sendra et al., 2023; Sosnowy, 2014; Stage et al., 2024). In line with Sosnowy (2014), we argue that these changes democratize modern medicine while simultaneously generating a series of challenges that may represent a risk for public health in the long term, mostly centred around Erikainen et al.'s (2019) idea of responsibilization. Following this, the chapter closes by summarizing the ways in which digitalization has affected all levels of healthcare communication from the perspective of the care receiver and highlighting the importance of training in communication (Francés-Tecles & Camaño-Puig, 2024; Mather & Cummings, 2019) to better cope with the changes brought by this transformation.

The fourth chapter, "From the medical gaze to the digital gaze", investigates how modern medicine (Foucault, 1963/1994) has transformed into virtual medicine in the context of the digitalization of healthcare communication. Inspired by Foucault's (1963/1994) understanding of modern medicine, the chapter proceeds to unfold how the digitalization of disease changes the interaction between care providers and care receivers (Ritunga et al., 2024; Song et al., 2025; Tokuç & Varol, 2023), where the patient is no longer laying on a bed but is instead dispersed in the digital realm observed by a digital gaze that tries to follow signs of disease. The chapter further exposes the ways in which healthcare digitalization transforms both medical knowledge (i.e., medicine as a science) and medical practice (i.e., medicine as an art), where expertise is increasingly shared between care providers and care receivers rather than being solely retained by healthcare professionals (Ho, 2023; Hopstaken et al., 2021; Merrell, 2015; Song et al., 2025). In contrast to modern medicine (Foucault, 1963/1994), the chapter closes by arguing that the digitalization of disease allows for the respatialization and retemporalization of disease and its care, affecting not only medical practice but also other medical actions, such as healthcare professionals' education or the management of healthcare.

The fifth chapter, "Digitalization of sickness: Renegotiating health citizenship", delves into the final conflicted status of ill health in the triad of disease, illness, and sickness to highlight that being a patient in the eyes of society is now more complicated (Nordtug, 2021). The key point of the chapter revolves around the idea that the digitalization of healthcare communication has altered the power relationships between the state, the individual, and the market in ways where all these actors now have more authority to exercise their agency. Through a review of existing research on health citizenship and the ways in which the experience of being ill from the perspective of society operates, we show how the digitalization of healthcare communication has further polarized the relationship between empowerment and self-discipline (Henwood & Marent, 2019; Petrakaki et al., 2018, 2021), where the state and the market have more options to exercise medical social control and the patient has more power to challenge the experience of being ill from the perspective of society. We further expose how patients make use of the unlimited opportunities for self-care and health promotion that came along with the digitalization of healthcare communication for coping with the increasing pressures to meet the "moral obligation" of being well (Bagger et al., 2023; Klausen, 2024). The chapter concludes by emphasizing the importance of working towards a more balanced patienthood from the perspective of society.

We conclude this book by outlining once again its main contribution – the end of the (traditional) patient and the rise of a new sociocultural understanding of patienthood, where the digitalization of ill health can facilitate and weaken the empowerment of the patient simultaneously. We also outline how the changes in the communicative relations between care providers, care receivers, and healthcare organizations are manifested in the digital functions of healthcare, which in turn are altering the communication environment of healthcare communication and generating new communicative tasks for healthcare professionals.

Note

1 The WHO (1948, p. 1) defined "health" as "a state of complete physical, mental and social well-being and not merely the absence of disease or infirmity".

References

Aguerrebere, P. M., Pacanowski, T. G., & Matamoros, D. C. (2024). Hospitals' corporate communication initiatives during the Covid-19 outbreak: Experiences, challenges and future opportunities. *Observatorio (OBS*)*, *18*(2), 182–199. https://doi.org/10.15847/obsOBS18220242338

Alzghaibi, H. (2025). Healthcare practitioners' perceptions of mHealth application barriers: Challenges to adoption and strategies for enhancing digital health integration. *Healthcare*, *13*(5), 494. https://doi.org/10.3390/healthcare13050494

Andreassen, H. K., Dyb, K., May, C. R., Pope, C. J., & Warth, L. L. (2018). Digitized patient–provider interaction: How does it matter? A qualitative meta-synthesis. *Social Science & Medicine*, *215*, 36–44. https://doi.org/10.1016/j.socscimed.2018.08.036

Autio, L. (1980). Mitä vikaa on Baabelintalossa [What is wrong with the house of Babel]. *Sosiaalilääketieteellinen aikakauskirja*, *74*(5), 84–85.

Bagger, C., Einarsson, A. M., Alvarez, V. A., Klausen, M., & Lomborg, S. (2023). Digital resignation and the datafied welfare state. *Big Data & Society*, *10*(2). https://doi.org/10.1177/20539517231206806

Bosseldal, I. P. (2006, September 5). Värdelöst vetande i Babels hus [Worthless knowledge in the House of Babel]. *Göteborgs-Posten*. https://www.gp.se/kultur/vardelost-vetande-i-babels-hus.66511219–641f-49f3–92ed-b64d96e6abb7

Brennen, J. S., & Kreiss, D. (2016). Digitalization. In K. B. Jensen, E. W. Rothenbuhler, J. D. Pooley, & R. T. Craig (Eds.), *The international encyclopedia of communication theory and philosophy* (1st ed., pp. 1–11). Wiley. https://doi.org/10.1002/9781118766804.wbiect111

Britannica. (2025, March 3). *History of computing*. https://www.britannica.com/technology/computer/History-of-computing

Cao, B., & Wang, L. (2024). When epidemic outbreaks meet social media: Collective illness narratives on WeChat during COVID-19 Omicron infection in China. *Health Communication*, *39*(11), 2211–2224. https://doi.org/10.1080/10410236.2023.2259695

CDC. (2024, June 6). *One health history*. https://www.cdc.gov/one-health/about/one-health-history.html

Chidambaram, S., Jain, B., Jain, U., Mwavu, R., Baru, R., Thomas, B., Greaves, F., Jayakumar, S., Jain, P., Rojo, M., Battaglino, M. R., Meara, J. G., Sounderajah, V., Celi, L. A., & Darzi, A. (2024). An introduction to digital determinants of health. *PLoS Digital Health*, *3*(1), e0000346. https://doi.org/10.1371/journal.pdig.0000346

Choi, P. J., Oskouian, R. J., & Tubbs, R. S. (2018). Telesurgery: Past, present, and future. *Cureus*, *10*(5), e2716. https://doi.org/10.7759/cureus.2716

Costa, D. S. J., Mercieca-Bebber, R., Tesson, S., Seidler, Z., & Lopez, A.-L. (2019). Patient, client, consumer, survivor or other alternatives? A scoping review of preferred terms for labelling individuals who access healthcare across settings. *BMJ Open*, *9*(3), e025166. https://doi.org/10.1136/bmjopen-2018-025166

Curtis, F., & Gillen, J. (2019). "I don't see myself as a 40-year-old on Facebook": Medical students' dilemmas in developing professionalism with social media. *Journal of Further and Higher Education*, *43*(2), 251–262. https://doi.org/10.1080/0309877X.2017.1359503

Dutta, M. J. (2008). *Communicating health: A culture-centered approach*. Polity Press.

Dutta, M. J. (2010). The critical cultural turn in *Health Communication*: Reflexivity, solidarity, and praxis. *Health Communication*, *25*(6–7), 534–539. https://doi.org/10.1080/10410236.2010.497995

Dussauge, I. (2004). Questioning medical technology: The discourse on technology in Läkartidningen 1978–1985. *Polhem*, *1*, 65–89.

EFSA. (2024, December 10). *Animal health*. https://www.efsa.europa.eu/en/topics/topic/animal-health

Erikainen, S., Pickersgill, M., Cunningham-Burley, S., & Chan, S. (2019). Patienthood and participation in the digital era. *Digital Health*, *5*. https://doi.org/10.1177/2055207619845546

Eriksson-Backa, K., Ahmad, F., Huvila, I., Enwald, H., & Hirvonen, N. (2022). Everyday health information literacy and attitudes towards digital health services among Finnish older adults. In S. Kurbanoglu, S. Spiranec, Y. Ünal, J. Boustany, & D. Kos (Eds.), *Information literacy in a post-truth era – ECIL 2021* (pp. 314–325). Springer. https://doi.org/10.1007/978-3-030-99885-1_27

Fiammenghi, C., Covolo, L., Vanoncini, A., Gelatti, U., & Ceretti, E. (2024). Institutional health communication and social media: Exploring Italian hospitals' use of social media pages. *Digital Health*, *10*. https://doi.org/10.1177/20552076241245921

Fleischer, S., Berg, A., Zimmermann, M., Wüste, K., & Behrens, J. (2009). Nurse-patient interaction and communication: A systematic literature review. *Journal of Public Health*, *17*(5), 339–353. https://doi.org/10.1007/s10389-008-0238-1

Flores-Sandoval, C., Sibbald, S., Ryan, B. L., & Orange, J. B. (2021). Healthcare teams and patient-related terminology: A review of concepts and uses. *Scandinavian Journal of Caring Sciences*, *35*(1), 55–66. https://doi.org/10.1111/scs.12843

Foucault, M. (1994). *The birth of the clinic: An archaeology of medical perception*. Vintage Books. (Original work published 1963)

Francés-Tecles, E., & Camaño-Puig, R. (2024). Experiencia y percepción de las enfermeras respecto del proceso de comunicación con los pacientes [Experience and perceptions of nurses regarding the communication process with patients]. *Revista de Comunicación y Salud*, *14*, 1–15. https://doi.org/10.35669/rcys.2024.14.e342

Frumkin, H. (2016). Introduction to environmental health. In H. Frumkin (Ed.), *Environmental health: From global to local* (3rd ed., pp. 58–91). Jossey-Bass.

Gavrilov, G., Simov, O., & Trajkovik, V. (2020). Analysis of digitalization in healthcare: Case study. In V. Dimitrova & I. Dimitrovski (Eds.), *ICT innovations 2020. Machine learning and applications* (pp. 202–216). Springer. https://doi.org/10.1007/978-3-030-62098-1_17

Gonzalez-Polledo, E. (2016). Chronic media worlds: Social media and the problem of pain communication on tumblr. *Social Media + Society*, *2*(1), 1–11. https://doi.org/10.1177/2056305116628887

Gonzalez-Polledo, E., & Tarr, J. (2016). The thing about pain: The remaking of illness narratives in chronic pain expressions on social media. *New Media & Society*, *18*(8), 1455–1472. https://doi.org/10.1177/1461444814560126

Guidry, J. P. D., Meganck, S. L., Lovari, A., Messner, M., Medina-Messner, V., Sherman, S., & Adams, J. (2020). Tweeting about #Diseases and #Publichealth: Communicating global health issues across nations. *Health Communication*, *35*(9), 1137–1145. https://doi.org/10.1080/10410236.2019.1620089

Gybel Jensen, C., Gybel Jensen, F., & Loft, M. I. (2024). Patients' experiences with digitalization in the health care system: Qualitative interview study. *Journal of Medical Internet Research*, *26*, e47278. https://doi.org/10.2196/47278

Ha, J. F., & Longnecker, N. (2010). Doctor–patient communication: A review. *The Ochsner Journal*, *10*(1), 38–43. https://pmc.ncbi.nlm.nih.gov/articles/PMC3096184/

Hall, D. (Creator). (2022). *Baymax!* [TV series]. Walt Disney Animation Studios & Walt Disney Pictures.

Hall, D., & Williams, C. (Directors). (2014). *Big Hero 6* [Film]. Walt Disney Animation Studios & Walt Disney Pictures.

Henwood, F., & Marent, B. (2019). Understanding digital health: Productive tensions at the intersection of sociology of health and science and technology studies. *Sociology of Health & Illness*, *41*(S1), 1–15. https://doi.org/10.1111/1467-9566.12898

Ho, A. (2023). Artificial intelligence as a feminist bioethics issue. In W. A. Rogers, J. L. Scully, S. M. Carter, V. A. Entwistle, & C. Mills (Eds.), *The Routledge Handbook of Feminist Bioethics* (pp. 291–307). Routledge.

Hogg, C. (1999). *Patients, power and politics: From patients to citizens*. SAGE Publications.

Hopstaken, J. S., Verweij, L., Van Laarhoven, C. J. H. M., Blijlevens, N. M. A., Stommel, M. W. J., 6 Hermens, R. P. M. G. (2021). Effect of digital care platforms on quality of care for oncological patients and barriers and facilitators for their implementation: Systematic review. *Journal of Medical Internet Research*, *23*(9), e28869. https://doi.org/10.2196/28869

Huber, M., Knottnerus, J. A., Green, L., Van der Horst, H., Jadad, A. R., Kromhout, D., Leonard, B., Lorig, K., Loureiro, M. I., Van der Meer, J. W. M., Schnabel, P., Smith, R., Van Weel, C., & Smid, H. (2011). How should we define health?. *BMJ*, *343*, d4163. https://doi.org/10.1136/bmj.d4163

Iyawa, G. E., Herselman, M., & Botha, A. (2016). Digital health innovation ecosystems: From systematic literature review to conceptual framework. *Procedia Computer Science*, *100*, 244–252. https://doi.org/10.1016/j.procs.2016.09.149

Jackson, S. (2023). Online health communities in controversy over ME/CFS and long Covid. *European Journal of Health Communication*, *4*(2), 49–72. https://doi.org/10.47368/ejhc.2023.203

Jersild, P. C. (1982). Babels hus efterspelet [House of Babel aftermath]. *Socialmedicinsk Tidskrift*, *59*(7–8), 320–323.

Jersild, P. C. (1987). *House of Babel*. University of Nebraska Press.

Jovy-Klein, F., Stead, S., Salge, T. O., Sander, J., Diehl, A., & Antons, D. (2024). Forecasting the future of smart hospitals: Findings from a real-time Delphi study. *BMC Health Services Research*, *24*, 1421. https://doi.org/10.1186/s12913-024-11895-z

Klausen, M. (2024). Disconnective care: Chronic illness and digital patienthood. In K. Albris, K. Fast, F. Karlsen, A. Kaun, S. Lomborg, & T. Syvertsen (Eds.), *The digital backlash and the paradoxes of disconnection* (pp. 153–170). Nordicom. https://doi.org/10.48335/9789188855961-8

Lefrançois, T., Malvy, D., Atlani-Duault, L., Benamouzing, D., Druais, P., Yazdanpanah, Y., Delfraissy, J., & Lina, B. (2023). After 2 years of the COVID-19 pandemic, translating One Health into action is urgent. *The Lancet*, *401*(10378), 789–794. https://doi.org/10.1016/S0140-6736(22)01840–2

Lupton, D. (1995). *The imperative of health: Public health and the regulated body*. SAGE Publications.

Lupton, D. (2013). The digitally engaged patient: Self-monitoring and self-care in the digital health era. *Social Theory & Health*, *11*(3), 256–270. https://doi.org/10.1057/sth.2013.10

Lupton, D. (2022a). *COVID societies: Theorising the coronavirus crisis*. Routledge.

Lupton, D. (2022b). From human-centric digital health to digital one health: Crucial new directions for mutual flourishing. *Digital Health*, *8*. https://doi.org/10.1177/20552076221129103

Maaß, L., Zeeb, H., & Rothgang, H. (2024). International perspectives on measuring national digital public health system maturity through a multidisciplinary Delphi study. *npj Digital Medicine*, *7*, 92. https://doi.org/10.1038/s41746-024-01078-9

Mather, C. A., & Cummings, E. (2019). Developing and sustaining digital professionalism: A model for assessing readiness of healthcare environments and capability of nurses. *BMJ Health & Care Informatics*, *26*(1), e100062. https://doi.org/10.1136/bmjhci-2019-100062

McCartney, G., Popham, F., McMaster, R., & Cumbers, A. (2019). Defining health and health inequalities. *Public Health*, *172*, 22–30. https://doi.org/10.1016/j.puhe.2019.03.023

Merrell, R. C. (2015). Geriatric telemedicine: Background and evidence for telemedicine as a way to address the challenges of geriatrics. *Healthcare Informatics Research*, *21*(4), 223–229. https://doi.org/10.4258/hir.2015.21.4.223

Merriam-Webster. (n.d.). *Patient*. Merriam-Webster.com Dictionary. Retrieved January 24, 2025, from https://www.merriam-webster.com/dictionary/patient

Nordin, G., & Ljungström, M. (2021, January 25). Huddinge sjukhus – lika stort som Gamla stan [Huddinge Hospital – as big as the Old Town]. *Locum*. https://www.locum.se/om-oss/press/nyheter/2021/huddinge-sjukhus-historia/

Nordtug, M. (2021). Who knows best? Health risks and digital media engagement in discourses relating to human papillomavirus vaccination. *Sociology of Health & Illness*, *43*(5), 1191–1205. https://doi.org/10.1111/1467-9566.13284

Ohia, C. M. D., & Uwalaka, E. C. (2021). Covid 19: A call to one health action. *Annals of Ibadan Postgraduate Medicine*, *19*(Sup. 1), S31–S37. https://pmc.ncbi.nlm.nih.gov/articles/PMC8791397/

Oxford English Dictionary. (n.d.). *Patient*. OED.com Dictionary. Retrieved January 24, 2024, from https://www.oed.com/dictionary/patient_adj?tl=true

Petrakaki, D., Hilberg, E., & Waring, J. (2018). Between empowerment and self-discipline: Governing patients' conduct through technological self-care. *Social Science & Medicine*, *213*, 146–153. https://doi.org/10.1016/j.socscimed.2018.07.043

Petrakaki, D., Hillberg, E., & Waring, J. (2021). The cultivation of digital health citizenship. *Social Science & Medicine*, *270*, 113675. https://doi.org/10.1016/j.socscimed.2021.113675

Ressler, P. K., Bradshaw, Y. S., Gualtieri, L., & Chui, K. K. H. (2012). Communicating the experience of chronic pain and illness through blogging. *Journal of Medical Internet Research*, *14*(5), e143. https://doi.org/10.2196/jmir.2002

Ritunga, I., Claramita, M., Widaty, S., & Soebono, H. (2024). Challenges and recommendations in the implementation of audiovisual telemedicine communication: A systematic review. *Korean Journal of Medical Education, 36*(3), 315–326. https://doi.org/10.3946/kjme.2024.305

Scott, R. (Director). (2012). *Prometheus* [Film]. 20th Century Studios.

Sendra, A. (2019). *Health communication processes in social media: Towards a transformative intervention on the information about chronic pain* [Doctoral dissertation, Universitat Rovira i Virgili]. Tesis Doctorals en Xarxa.

Sendra, A., & Farré, J. (2017). Institutional pain communication via Twitter by Spanish and US pain societies: Analysis of levels of use and engagement. *Catalan Journal of Communication & Cultural Studies*, *9*(1), 3–23. https://doi.org/10.1386/cjcs.9.1.3_1

Sendra, A., & Farré, J. (2020). Communicating the experience of chronic pain through social media: Patients' narrative practices on Instagram. *Journal of Communication in Healthcare*, *13*(1), 46–54. https://doi.org/10.1080/17538068.2020.1752982

Sendra, A., Torkkola, S., & Parviainen, J. (2023). Non-knowledge in medical practices: Approaching the uses of social media in healthcare from an epistemological perspective. *Journal of Digital Social Research*, *5*(1), 70–89. https://doi.org/10.33621/jdsr.v5i1.152

Sevilä, A. (1980). Vavahduttava tarina suursairaalan elämästä [A startling story of life in a major hospital]. *Syöpä*, *5*, 22–24.

Sharf, B. F., & Street Jr, R. L. (1997). The patient as a central construct: Shifting the emphasis. *Health Communication*, *9*(1), 1–11. https://doi.org/10.1207/s15327027hc0901_1

Smith, R. (2008, July 8). Richard Smith: The end of disease and the beginning of health. *BMJ Opinion*. https://blogs.bmj.com/bmj/2008/07/08/richard-smith-the-end-of-disease-and-the-beginning-of-health/

Song, M., Elson, J., & Bastola, D. (2025). Digital age transformation in patient-physician communication: 25-year narrative review (1999–2023). *Journal of Medical Internet Research*, *27*, e60512. https://doi.org/10.2196/60512

Sontag, S. (2002). *Illness as metaphor*. Penguin.

Sosnowy, C. (2014). Practicing patienthood online: Social media, chronic illness, and lay expertise. *Societies*, *4*(2), 316–329. https://doi.org/10.3390/soc4020316

Stage, C., Karlsson, A., & Ledderer, L. (2024). Online patient work: On the use of peer-led online communities to process and prevent discontinuity of care. *European Journal of Health Communication*, *5*(2), 44–59. https://doi.org/10.47368/ejhc.2024.203

Svensson, C. (2024, March 23). Babels hus [House of Babel]. *Presskraft*. https://presskraft.se/babels-hus/

Tokuç, B., & Varol, G. (2023). Medical education in the era of advancing technology. *Balkan Medical Journal*, *40*(6), 395–399. https://doi.org/10.4274/balkanmedj.galenos.2023.2023-7-79

Torkkola, S., Tyni, P., Parviainen, J., & Sendra, A. (2024). Terveydenhuollon muuttuvat viestintäkäytännöt: Kyselytutkimus terveydenhuollon asiantuntijoille sosiaalisen median mahdollisuuksista ja uhista potilastyössä [Changing practices in healthcare communication: A survey for healthcare experts about opportunities and threats of social media in patient care]. *Media & Viestintä, 47*(4), 53–78. https://doi.org/10.23983/mv.130759

Vaagan, R. W., Torkkola, S., Sendra, A., Farré, J., & Lovari, A. (2021). A critical analysis of the digitization of healthcare communication in the EU: A comparison of Italy, Finland, Norway, and Spain. *International Journal of Communication, 15*, 1718–1740. https://ijoc.org/index.php/ijoc/article/view/15399

Whedon, J., Whedon, J., & Tancharoen, M. (Creators). (2013–2020). *Agents of S.H.I.E.L.D* [TV series]. ABC Signature, Marvel Television & Mutant Enemy Productions.

WHO. (n.d.). *One Health*. https://www.who.int/health-topics/one-health

WHO. (1948). *Constitution of the World Health Organization*. http://apps.who.int/gb/bd/PDF/bd47/EN/constitution-en.pdf?ua=1

WHO. (2023). *Classification of digital interventions, services and applications in health: A shared language to describe the uses of digital technology for health* (2nd ed.). World Health Organization.

2 Communication and ill health

In this chapter, we focus on understanding health communication and discuss how the concept of health communication has been defined. Furthermore, we consider how the connection between communication and ill health has been understood. In the field, there is no common understanding of what health communication is or what its relation is to ill health (Torkkola, 2016). A clear definition of healthcare communication is almost entirely lacking. The recently published *International Encyclopedia of Health Communication* (Ho et al., 2023) reflects this state of deprivation: a definition of healthcare communication is not included, and a definition of health communication is also lacking in the encyclopaedia. One possible reason for not defining these concepts springs from the diversity of health communication scholars as well as their mostly practically oriented research tasks. Health communication is a crossroads where scholars and practitioners from multifaceted backgrounds, practices, and aims meet and cooperate (Kreps, 2020; Torkkola, 2016).

There are two questions that must be addressed for the open understanding of health communication: which sub-fields of communication are included in health communication, and how the connection between communication and ill health is apprehended? In the field of media and communication studies, there are plenty of different typologies of communication: some of them are driven by the empirical area of the studies and some by the theoretical model of communication (Helles, 2016). The digitalization of communication has increased the diversity of communication, and even many of these new extensions of communication can be seen as a transformation of previous genres of communication (Helles, 2016; Jensen & Helles, 2011). In the field of health communication, there is diversity of the same kind. For example, the papers presented in the health communication sessions of the IAMCR and NordMedia conferences cover digital and non-digital communication, interpersonal communication, journalism, mass communication, media communication, and even organizational communication. Over the last decades, the understanding of the area of health communication has changed, too. At the beginning of the 1970s, health communication was launched under the name "therapeutic communication" and understood as interpersonal communication (Kreps et al., 1998,

DOI: 10.4324/9781003519607-2

p. 8). Therapeutic communication is suited only to scholars who are oriented to interpersonal communication. Therefore, the broader concept of health communication, consisting of mass communication, health campaigns, and organization as well as interpersonal communication, replaced the term therapeutic communication (Kreps et al., 1998). However, there is no consensus on what kind of communication is included within health communication. The definitions of health communication by the WHO (1998, 2021) are among the best known and used definitions. According to the earlier definition (WHO, 1998), health communication consists only of mass communication, while the latter one (WHO, 2021) includes all forms of communication. Today, the broader definition of health communication, including all forms and channels of communication, seems to be dominant (Thomas, 2010; Viswanathan, 2008).

Nowadays, there are also several sub-fields of communication in which researchers are interested, and studies have been conducted at the individual, interpersonal, social network, organizational, and mass or societal levels (Viswanathan, 2008). For us, health communication is

> a multidisciplinary and versatile field of study that, using both traditional and new communication processes, aims to improve (through promotion, literacy, and education) (1) the interactions between all the stakeholders who take part of the health system (either citizens, patients, health professionals or organizations at different levels); and (2) the quality, efficiency, and management of health and malady (as individuals) and of the health care system (as a society).
>
> (Sendra, 2019, pp. 41–42)

Malady here is understood as ill health (see further discussion below). Following this wide understanding of the health communication research field, we see all communication addressing health and illness in some way as health communication; thus, ill health is communicated and constructed in all forms and channels of communication – i.e., interpersonal communication, mass communication, and organizational communication (Torkkola, 2016). We see healthcare communication as a sub-field of health communication consisting of all communicative actions between its members and collaborators (Figure 2.1).

Organizational communication scholars understand communication as a constituent part of the organization, but it is not solely a constituent part (Bisel, 2010; Putnam et al., 2009). According to Putnam et al. (2009, p. 4), the communicative constitution of organizations (CCO) "presumably embodies the material (composition or elements), the formal (framing or forming), and the efficient causes (principles or rules for governing) that bring organizations into existence". Robert D. McPhee and Pamela Zaug (2000) view CCO as consisting of four types of constituting communication processes, which they call "flows". The four flows involve the processes of membership negotiation,

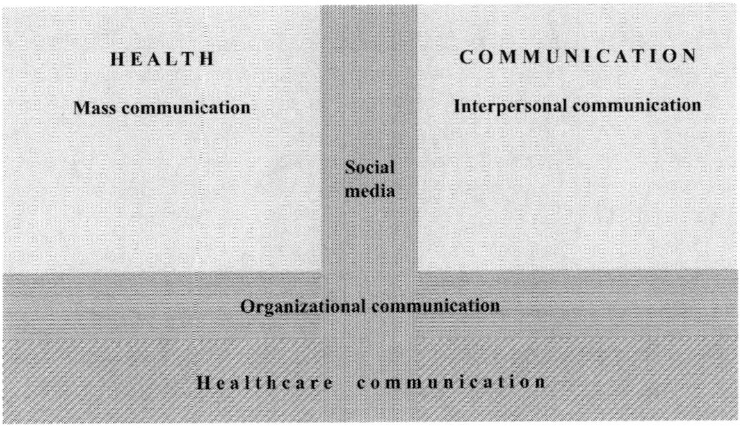

Figure 2.1 Types of health communication.[1] Created by the authors.

organizational self-structuring, activity coordination, and institutional positioning (McPhee & Zaug, 2000). Organizational communication as a discursive practice rooted in particular social structures engages members of the organization in power relations (Deetz & Mumby, 1990). Stanley Deetz and Dennis K. Mumby (1990, p. 41) argue that "discourse is both medium and product of the power relations that characterize organizational behavior". Following the organizational communication scholars, we see healthcare communication as an essential condition of the organization. The communicative actions invite the members of the healthcare organization into a certain institutional position that frames their actions as a provider or receiver of healthcare services. That framing can be both empowering and restricting.

Healthcare communication includes both mass and interpersonal communication, where communication acts could be messages from one to one, one to many, or many to many (Jensen & Helles, 2011). The digitalization of healthcare changes communication not only between the care provider and care receiver but also within institution–institution, institution–patient, provider–institution, patient–institution, patient–provider, and patient–patient relationships (Vaagan et al., 2021). The digitalization of healthcare communication digitalizes ill health and care and invites the reconstruction of health professionalism and patienthood. Table 2.1 gathers together the topics communicated by institutions, care providers, and care receivers.

Healthcare communication utilizes all forms of communication, and the digitalization of healthcare communication is driven by all of this communication. Interpersonal communication is based on face-to-face interaction between a care provider and care receiver or between other healthcare experts and healthcare service users. It includes traditional forms of communication, like

Table 2.1 Topics of communication in healthcare communication (reviewed from Torkkola, 2018)

	Institution (healthcare centres, hospitals, and health authorities)	*Care provider (healthcare professionals, doctors, and nurses)*	*Care receiver (patients, clients, and citizens)*
Institution	medical recording, service management and allocation, decision-making	work induction and management	information on healthcare services, self-care, and health promotion
Care provider	practices of services, medical recording	consultation, collegial support	medical examination, anamnesis, health advice
Care receiver	information and feedback on healthcare services, advice seeking on illness care and health promotion	advice seeking on illness care and health promotion, feedback on received care	sharing information and experience on illness care, health promotion, and healthcare services, peer support

oral communication and written correspondence, and new forms of communication, like digital platforms, that facilitate both simultaneous and separate interactions. In mass communication, information is sent to all collaborators and citizens. To deliver that information, both traditional media, like printed leaflets, magazines, or television and radio advertising, and new media, like social media and Internet pages owned by the organization itself or another public organization, can be used.

Journalism as the fourth estate has been seen as central to pluralist democratic processes promoting and facilitating public discussion (Dutton, 2009) that may lead to changes in society, including healthcare (see, e.g., Motamedi et al., 2023). Today, the authority of journalism is being challenged by new media, called the fifth estate by William H. Dutton (2009). The delivery of information also includes dis- and misinformation that is not shared by the organization itself. This kind of information delivered from outside the organization could appear accidentally or be shared deliberately to harm the organization (Sendra et al., 2024). The information on healthcare could be based on information delivered by the organization itself but also on information sources found by journalists, including information leaked from within the organization by personnel or patients. For example, the International Consortium of Investigative Journalists, with more than 250 journalists from 36 countries, analysed over eight million device-related health records, including death and injury reports and recalls, and revealed the harm caused by medical devices that have been tested inadequately or not at all (ICIJ, n.d.).

2.1 Communicating ill health

The second question about defining health communication concerns the relation between communication and ill health. In the field of health communication studies, the relation between communication and ill health has been understood in dissimilar, even conflicting, ways (Torkkola, 2016). Browner (1999, p. 138) describes this disparity by quoting Linda Hut's remark based on her dream about sitting at a conference table and arguing with a group of frustrated physicians: "If it looks like a duck, walks like a duck, and quacks like a duck, it's a duck! One shouted. Equally frustrated, I shouted back: What do you mean by a duck?". Because of this diversity and conflicting understanding, we see that it is more important than ever to outline how we understand health communication and what differences or connections it has to other implicit or explicit understandings of communication.

In contrast to the communication sciences, the cultural turn (Pietilä, 2005, pp. 255–272) has stayed on the margins of health communication, where most studies have adopted a practical orientation. This practical orientation is manifested in health communication textbooks (e.g., Cross et al., 2017; Thomas, 2010; Wright et al., 2008), which focus on the largely instrumental use of communication in health promotion and illness care. Similarly, most of the health communication research has focused on analysing the impact of health promotion campaigns by measuring health behaviour changes or determining the accuracy of health messages spread in the media (Torkkola, 2016). Among researchers, there has been a long debate on the efficacy of mediated health campaigns (Snyder et al., 2004, p. 72), and discussion on the valid methods to measure the efficacy of health campaigns continues (Anker et al., 2016; Noar et al., 2009, 2020).

Among culturally oriented health communication scholars, such as Deborah Lupton (see, e.g., 1995, 2003) and Mohan Dutta (2008, 2010), there have been more critical discussions on the efficacy of health campaigns. The understanding of health communication as a linear process where health messages are carried from the sender to the receiver over a channel is seen as problematic in many ways (Lupton, 1995, pp. 106–114). Furthermore, according to this linear understanding of health communication, people have been seen as a passive target group and not active message decoding readers with multiple cultural and social backgrounds interpreting and using messages from their own perspectives and for their own purposes. Understanding the use of health and medical information cannot be based solely on the analysis of texts; it requires an analysis of how people themselves interpret and use said texts. In an analysis of the reception of medical dramas, Davin (2003, p. 673, emphasis in original) points out the audience's ability to simultaneously have two incompatible viewing modes: "cognitive *and* emotional, distant *and* involved, informing *and* enjoying themselves".

The critical discussion focuses not only on the problem of the efficacy of health communication but also on understanding health communication itself.

Since the beginning of the 1990s, there has been critical discussion in the field of health communication on the understanding of health communication, particularly on the relations between communication and ill health (Dutta, 2010; Lupton, 1994, 1995, pp. 106–114). This critical discussion challenges the instrumental understanding of health communication and value-free medicine and opens the discussion on how biomedical hegemony, as a part of power structures, can cover ill health as a socially and culturally constructed entity.

Even if the critical discussion and culturally oriented approach are today more present within the field of health communication, in practice, communication is seen mostly instrumentally and not as a part of the entity of ill health. Most health communication actors are not familiar with the perspectives of communication and social science. The authors have faced this biomedical hegemony in the teaching of health communication to students of medicine and health sciences. One of us, Sinikka Torkkola, has tried to overcome this hegemony by starting lectures by showing a nondescript picture (see an example of these pictures in Figure 2.2) to students and asking their opinion about it. Before answering the question, the students start to guess what the picture is about, naming it, which follows a discussion on how we need to name an object before even beginning to discuss it. Typically, the discussion then continues by explaining that, although outside of language, there probably are some states

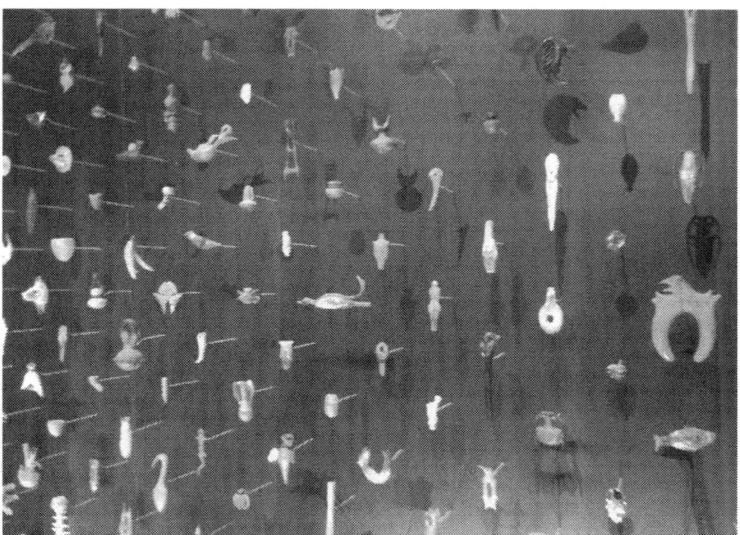

Figure 2.2 Example of a nondescript picture used in the lectures with students.[2] The image has been converted to greyscale for the purposes of this publication. Photograph by Sinikka Torkkola (2018).

of being that we could call health, illness, or something in between, we cannot speak with those states of being without language and naming. The discussion about the nondescript picture opens up the question of the relationship between communication and ill health and gets us to see communication not instrumentally but as a part of the entity of ill health. The discussion also opens up the question of the possibility of transdisciplinary discussion. German philosopher Hans-George Gadamer, in his lecture *Philosophy and Medicine* in Heidelberg in 1989 (Naukkarinen, 2004), stated that in science there still exists one common, indisputable domain – language – in which "experience and knowledge become sedimented and speak directly to us through the words themselves" (Gadamer, 1993, p. 122, 1996, p. 93).

Following Gadamer's view, we see that there is an opportunity to understand altered viewpoints and acknowledge the diversity of ill health. This is essential for this book, too. To understand the construction of ill health in multiple communication actions in healthcare, we need to see the differences between illnesses communicated by institutions, care providers, physicians, and nurses, and care receivers, patients, customers, and citizens. All of them have special viewpoints on ill health and different ways to communicate it, but furthermore, illness, disease, and sickness are also part of a human existence that is much more diverse than simply being or not being ill.

2.2 Communicating health and illness

For us, health communication is based on a perspective of communication as a cultural phenomenon maintaining, producing, and transforming health and illnesses. Health communication is not only the mediation or transmission of health and illness messages from the sender to the receiver; it also produces health and illness (Torkkola, 2016). This production does not mean that health and illnesses in health communication are not related to other textual and non-textual health and illnesses, but rather, they are a part of the sociocultural entity of health and illnesses (Torkkola, 2016).

In healthcare, the communicative actions springing from the tasks of caring for illness and promoting health and communication are comparable to other instruments of care, such as medication or surgery (Eskola & Puustinen, 1996). This instrumental orientation invites us to focus on communicative practices, communication channels, and the skills of communicators. In this book, we want to see beyond this instrumental understanding of communication and think about communication as a part of a healthcare entity where ill health, health professionalism, and patienthood are constructed in healthcare communication.

The culturally centred health communication approach offers an alternative to the biomedical model of ill health. Fundamental to the culture-centred approach is the understanding that communication about health involves the negotiation of shared meanings embedded in socially constructed identities, relationships, social norms, and structures (Dutta, 2008, pp. 44–45, 55). Thus, there is no health and illness per se; there are different temporal and spatial conditions directing what kind of individual and collective statuses are experienced or delineated as health or not health. The theoretical and methodological challenge of this book (and more generally in health communication) is to determine how to generate a cultural understanding in practice, how to see the plurality of ill health, and how to dismantle biomedical hegemony.

Against this background, we need to take a closer look at the concept of ill health. On the one hand, there is no coherent understanding of the concept of ill health, and many kinds of concepts under the category of human ailment are connected to it. These include "disease", "malady", "defects", "disability", "handicap", "deformity", "disfigurement", "infirmity", "impairment", "dysfunction", "dystrophy", "abnormality", "debility", "derangement", "malignancy", "morbidity", "suffering", "pain", "weakness", "incompetence", "illness", "sickness", "symptom", and "syndrome" (Hofmann, 2001, p. 224). On the other hand, and in contrast to the English language, in other European languages, there is no distinction between the words "ill" and "sick". When Andrew Twaddle (1994) wrote about the triad of disease, illness, and sickness in Swedish, he did not use Swedish but the English words disease, illness, and sickness. This paucity of vocabulary became evident too when one of us, Sinikka Torkkola, wrote a book of her dissertation titled *Sick Story: Research on Theory of Health Journalism and the Newspaper Hospital* (Torkkola, 2008). She suggested the use of a new Finnish word – "potemus" – for illness, but it remained only an attempt, as it has not been taken up. As far as we know, the distinction is not made in other European languages either, such as Catalan, German, Russian, or Spanish.

With the aim of getting out of this jungle of concepts, we need to ask from which perspective these concepts are used. In the context of healthcare communication, we can see three different dimensions, namely medicine, experience, and society, which are manifested in different concepts of human ailment: disease, illness, and sickness. The distinction between disease, illness, and sickness was first elaborated by the sociologist Andrew Twaddle in his 1967 dissertation (Hofmann, 2016, p. 16). The distinction between disease, illness, and sickness has been largely expanded in medical sociology and anthropology ever since, but it has also been fundamentally challenged (Hofmann, 2002).

Lennart Nordenfelt (Twaddle & Nordenfelt, 1994, pp. 34–35) criticizes Twaddle's triad by outlining that it does not encompass the whole phenomenon of health and unhealth. For example, injury, impairment, defect, and disability are not included in the triad. Furthermore, Nordenfelt (Twaddle & Nordenfelt, 1994) debates whether there are two ideas mixed in the category of sickness: a social category with rights and duties and a deviant behaviour observed by others. He also points out that "there is no 'natural course of events' in which sickness is placed" (Twaddle & Nordenfelt, 1994, p. 35). Finally, he suggests

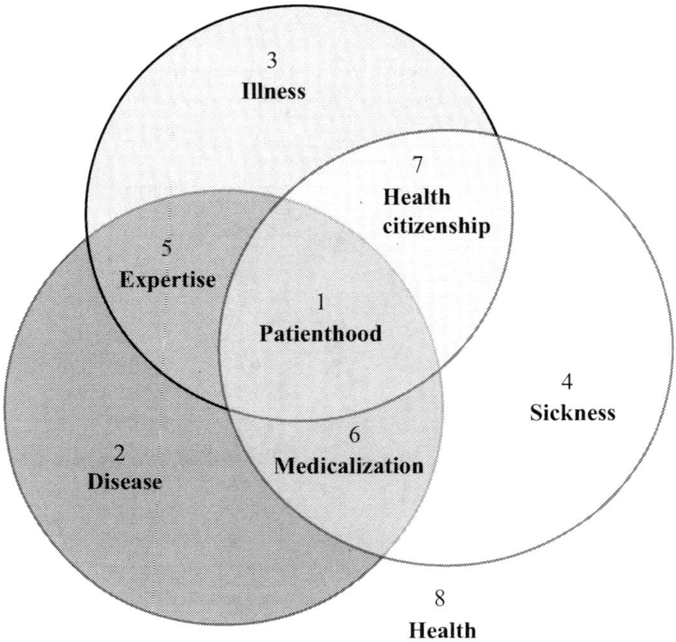

Figure 2.3 Dimensions of ill health.[3] Created by the authors.

that the triad should be completed by the general theory of health (Twaddle & Nordenfelt, 1994).

Figure 2.3 describes all statuses of a person being ill or well, diagnosed as diseased or not, and having the status of sick or not. In healthcare, the most usual case is patienthood (1), when a person feels ill, has a diagnosed disease, and possesses the social status of sick. Health (8) concerns the person who is well in all dimensions. The other dimensions of ill health, where a person could be at the same time ill in one dimension and well in another, are conflicting. These dimensions, denominated as expertise (5), medicalization (6), and health citizenship (7), are not labelled in previous triads (Hofmann, 2002, 2016; Torkkola, 2008; Twaddle & Nordenfelt, 1994), but they were designated thus in the writing of this book.

Historically, the word "disease" refers to the impediment of free movement; dis-ease is derived from the Old French and literally means the absence of ease or elbow room (Boyd, 2000). Disease, as we understand it today, is based on modern medicine and its birth in the eighteenth century, when treating illness became a modern science (Foucault, 1963/1994). Underlying the objective understanding of disease is the naturalistic definition of disease, as in the model defined by Boorse (1976); medical care is no longer targeted at the sick person but instead at the disease the person is carrying. With the advent of modern medicine, disease became the object of knowing instead of an object of treatment. The symptoms of an illness came to be interpreted as signs of disease; on this basis, the clinical gaze could find the abnormalities in the body (Foucault, 1963/1994, pp. 3–20). For modern medicine, disease is the (biological) manifestation of objective reality found in diagnosis, and the existence of disease is not dependent on human understanding (Wulff et al., 1990, pp. 79–82). In his definition of disease, Andrew Twaddle (Twaddle & Nordenfelt, 1994, p. 7) follows modern medicine and classifies disease as a "physiological malfunction: infection, mechanical breakdown, or degeneration resulting in reduced capacity and/or life expectancy". Bjørn Hofmann (2016, p. 230) has analysed the concept of disease and concluded that "[d]isease is a complex concept, that is, it has a complex extension, and does not lend itself to a simple definition". However, following Twaddle, we understand disease in the same way as Zsuzsanna Chappell, who summarizes the concept of disease as "pathological processes, seen in the medical gaze and communicated through a diagnosis" (Chappell, 2023, p. 79).

In the definition of illness by Twaddle (Twaddle & Nordenfelt, 1994, p. 7), illness is described as the "subjective definition of health status based on state perceptions and/or feelings of competence". Moreover, illness expresses emotions such as anxiety, fear, pain, and suffering and experience. In this sense, illness is subjective, and access to the illness experience of another person happens by verbalization (Hofmann, 2016). However, in contrast to Hofmann (2016), who limits illness communication to verbalization, we see that verbalization is only one method of communication for illness expression. A patient without the ability to deliver a vocal message, like a patient on mechanical ventilation in intensive care, could use other non-vocal methods, such as gestures, facial expressions, or other muscle movements, to express illness (Karlsen et al., 2023). Although illness is an individual experience, it is not constructed by the individual alone; instead, time and space set the conditions for individual ill-being, and illness is simultaneously subjective, intersubjective, and both culturally and societally constructed (Kleinman, 1988, pp. 4–30). Talcot Parsons' (1951) classic concept of the sick role, which refers to a patient's behaviour, is seen more contextually today, and patienthood is a cultural and social platform or frame that invites an ill person to be a patient (Lupton, 1993; Torkkola, 2008, pp. 219–220). Compared to the sick role, patienthood is a stage that invites a person to act as a patient.

The third dimension of ill health, sickness, is the social response to illness and disease. For Twaddle (Twaddle & Nordenfelt, 1994, p. 7), sickness is a "social definition based on identity in the eyes of others and/or social functioning". Sickness includes a wide range of informal and formal benefits and harms, such as access to treatment, sick pay, financial and social support, legitimate demands for rest, stigmatization, and discrimination (Chappell, 2023, pp. 80–81), and it involves expectations, conventions, policies, and social norms and roles as basic phenomena (Susser, 1990). Sickness determines the right to treatment and economic rights as well as legal accountability (Hofmann, 2016). However, sickness acts rarely by itself but in conjunction with disease, entitling access to treatment and social benefits (Hofmann, 2016, p. 211).

In expertise (5), a condition faces medical/expert and experience-based/experiential knowledge that conflicts with sickness. In conditions of this kind, a person feels ill and has been diagnosed with a disease but has not been defined as sick by society. For example, people feeling ill with a diagnosed disease will not get a disability pension if their application is rejected by the social insurance institution (Laaksonen et al., 2018). Expertise is understood as a social phenomenon, especially from a sociological and anthropological perspective (Eyal, 2019), where the generation of knowledge is impacted by the "social context, both social structure (the perceived regularities in the social network) and social knowledge" (Carley, 1986, p. 381). In other words, both care providers and care receivers generate knowledge within social structures and in interaction with others (Carley, 1986). As a result, medical/expert and experience-based/experiential knowledge sometimes also conflict with each other, as the social structures generating medical/expert knowledge enjoy a certain level of power that does not always welcome being questioned (Caron-Flinterman et al., 2005; Sendra et al., 2023). Experience-based/experiential knowledge has a record of "foregrounding the epistemic dimensions of personal experience, successfully influencing healthcare policy and biomedical research" (Mazanderani et al., 2020, p. 268). However, for that to happen, ideas not only need to circulate between care providers and care receivers (Arksey, 1994); communicative expertise (Sarangi, 2018) is also needed, which involves knowing both how to communicate your own knowledge and what the spaces are where the knowledge generated by others is being communicated. In the context of digitalization, experience-based/experiential knowledge is expected to have a determinant role in shaping the future of healthcare (Blume, 2017).

In medicalization (6), a person has been diagnosed with a disease and is defined as sick in the social order but does not feel ill. The involvement of medicine in the management of society is not seen to be new (Zola, 1972). Traditionally, medicalization has been described as a process by which non-medical problems become defined and treated as medical ones (Conrad, 1992). Hysteria (Showalter, 1998), drapetomania (Prasad, 2022), and the politically motivated psychiatric diagnosis of dissidents (Bonnie, 2002) are the classic examples of medicalization that manifest in the repression of the citizen by the state. However, medicalization is not merely a medical process but "a sociocultural process that may or may not involve the medical profession, lead to medical social control or medical treatment, or be the result of intentional expansion by the medical profession" (Conrad, 1992, p. 211). In addition to extreme repression by the medical and societal authorities, medicalization has also been understood as processes in which the phenomena of the human being become defined and treated as medical problems, like ageing (Saborido & García-Barranquero, 2022), childbirth (Al-Gailani & Davis, 2014), or deviant behaviour (Easterling, 2000). It is also possible to understand medicalization in conditions that happen during the medical consultation, where signs of disease like high blood pressure, pre-diabetes, or human papillomavirus (HPV) are found in laboratory tests or medical examinations even when a patient has not had an experience or symptoms of illness, and the patient receives a diagnosis of disease and perhaps also medication for it (Hofmann, 2016, p. 19).

Health citizenship (7) connects ill health and society. It is defined as a subcategory of social citizenship, which was first named at the beginning of the 1950s by Thomas Humphrey Marshall (2009) (see also Groleau, 2011; Harjula, 2015, p. 18). Mikko Jauho and Ilpo Helén (2023, p. 481) argue that "the concept of health citizenship is too restricted if it addresses health and illness as just a dimension of social citizenship". They understand health citizenship as citizenship by vitality that includes two dimensions of health citizenship: a membership (i.e., belonging to the organic unit of the nation-state) and an entitlement (i.e., the right of the individual citizen to healthcare) (Jauho & Helén, 2023). Health citizenship manifests itself also as an all-encompassing, penetrating call for citizens to behave in an increasingly healthier manner, which manifests "as a heightened sense of personal responsibility over one's own health and as more vocal blaming of those who are perceived as having failed to fulfil their obligation" (Jauho & Helén, 2023, p. 479). In the past, health promotion was a citizen's duty towards the nation and the state. Today, it is more persuasive (Jauho & Helén, 2023) and asks citizens not only to promote their own health but also to participate in the process of health knowledge production (Groleau, 2011, p. 815). In the triad of disease, illness, and sickness (Hofmann, 2016), the dimension of illness and sickness is described as a case where a person is ill and has the status of being sick but has not been diagnosed with a disease. Examples of cases of such a kind are chronic Lyme disease (Dumes, 2020) and medically unexplained symptoms (MUS) (Nettleton, 2006). These kinds of cases may not be so exceptional since, according to Aamland et al. (2012), medically unexplained physical symptoms (MUPS) have been a leading cause of sickness absence.

The dimensions of ill health are not clear-cut, on/off statuses of being, but fuzzy statuses overlapping each other (see, e.g., Sadegh-Zadeh, 2000), and only theoretically we see it as a definition of status of being. The purpose of Figure 2.3 is not to define ailments in individual cases but to help us to comprehend the prevailing cultural understanding of ill health and the hegemonic status of medicine and to see the multidimensionality of ill health. In the context of the digitalization of healthcare and its communication, it is essential that we see everywhere where ill health is communicated, not only those sites of healthcare taking centre stage.

2.3 Construction of patienthood in digital healthcare communication

The digitalization of healthcare has created both threats and desire. It has been perceived both as improving services and reducing their costs (Eden & Bloor, 2010; Neittaanmäki & Kaasalainen, 2018). However, for Jordi Piera-Jiménez et al. (2024, p. 16), the transition to digital healthcare services "is not just about adopting new technologies but also about a paradigm shift in healthcare delivery, moving from referrals and transferability of responsibility toward a collaboration emphasizing a holistic approach to patient care for improved health outcomes". In the digitalization of healthcare, communication is seen to play a key role in its success. Daniel Eden and Jonathan Bloor (2010, p. 114) argue that "communication in particular, plays a significant part in both the efficiency of an organization and the morale of its staff, with the success of the systems it has in place directly influencing" the provision of healthcare services.

The digitalization of healthcare alters not only communication practices but also patienthood, health professionalism, and ill health (Sendra et al., 2021). These communication practices are rooted in the sociocultural processes constructing ill health and occurring between the members and collaborators of the healthcare organization. Besides formal healthcare communication, there are countless communication actions concerning ill health and healthcare organizations. This informal communication can be viewed as "noise" that negatively affects organizational efficiency (Mumby, 2016). This noise is driven not only by communication within healthcare itself but also by the entity of the communication environment, which is described in the Introduction (see Figure 1.1). Moreover, communication that is evaluated as counterproductive or harmful noise by one actor could be evaluated as useful information by another. In a survey on Finnish hospital experts, every fifth respondent reported facing a conflict with a patient or a family member because of disinformation shared on social media or the Internet (Torkkola et al., 2024). Although this noisy information is harmful from the viewpoint of the doctor, for the patient, it could be useful and perhaps a source for empowerment, too. Concerning the respatialization of care driven by digital health, in future healthcare, the communication network will probably be denser and more widespread, and therefore noisier, which could increase conflicts between care providers and care receivers or, depending on the point of view, increase the empowerment of care receivers.

In this book, we focus on healthcare communication from the viewpoint of the patient, asking how patienthood is constructed in the communication of healthcare and how the digitalization of healthcare communication is altering patienthood. As we have pointed out in this chapter, patienthood as a sociocultural construction invites the ill person to be a patient in certain conditions that are rooted in the dimensions of ill health – i.e., disease, illness, and sickness – which are under reconstruction in the digitalization of healthcare organizations and, more generally, in the digitalization of ill health.

Notes

1 The sub-fields of health communication in the figure are not clear-cut or unchangeable forms or areas of health communication, but examples of the multifield communication concerning institutions and individuals (both professionals and lay people).

2 The *Artifact Panel* by William Morris works as an initiator for discussion on the relation between communication/language and ill health. The work is in the Portland Art Museum, Oregon (USA).

3 The triad of disease, illness, and sickness are dimensions of ill health and are based on figures by Twaddle (Twaddle & Nordenfelt, 1994), Hofmann (2002, 2016), and Torkkola (2008). Disease (2) could be seen as the medical or professional dimension of ailment, illness (3) as the individual or collective experience of ailment, and sickness (4) as the social order of ailment. Patienthood (1) and health (8) describe concurring statuses in every dimension of ill health. Expertise (5), medicalization (6), and health citizenship (7) describe the conflicted statuses of being ill.

References

Aamland, A., Malterud, K., & Werner, E. L. (2012). Phenomena associated with sick leave among primary care patients with medically unexplained physical symptoms: A systematic review. *Scandinavian Journal of Primary Health Care*, *30*(3), 147–155. https://doi.org/10.3109/02813432.2012.704812

Al-Gailani, S., & Davis, A. (2014). Introduction to "transforming pregnancy since 1900". *Studies in History and Philosophy of Science Part C: Studies in History and Philosophy of Biological and Biomedical Sciences*, *47*(Part B), 229–232. https://doi.org/10.1016/j.shpsc.2014.07.001

Anker, A. E., Feeley, T. H., McCracken, B., & Lagoe, C. A. (2016). Measuring the effectiveness of mass-mediated health campaigns through meta-analysis. *Journal of Health Communication*, *21*(4), 439–456. https://doi.org/10.1080/10810730.2015.1095820

Arksey, H. (1994). Expert and lay participation in the construction of medical knowledge. *Sociology of Health & Illness*, *16*(4), 448–468. https://doi.org/10.1111/1467-9566.ep11347516

Bisel, R. S. (2010). A communicative ontology of organization? A description, history, and critique of CCO theories for organization science. *Management Communication Quarterly*, *24*(1), 124–131. https://doi.org/10.1177/0893318909351582

Blume, S. (2017). In search of experiential knowledge. *Innovation: The European Journal of Social Science Research*, *30*(1), 91–103. https://doi.org/10.1080/13511610.2016.1210505

Bonnie, R. J. (2002). *Political abuse of psychiatry in the Soviet Union and in China: Complexities and controversies*. https://doi.org/10.2139/ssrn.1760001

Boorse, C. (1976). What a theory of mental health should be. *Journal for The Theory of Social Behavior*, *6*(1), 61–84. https://doi.org/10.1111/j.1468-5914.1976.tb00359.x

Boyd, K. M. (2000). Disease, illness, sickness, health, healing and wholeness: Exploring some elusive concepts. *Medical Humanities*, *26*(1), 9–17. https://doi.org/10.1136/mh.26.1.9

Browner, C. H. (1999). On the medicalisation of medical anthropology. *Medical Antropology Quarterly*, *13*(2), 135–140. https://www.jstor.org/stable/649641

Carley, K. (1986). Knowledge acquisition as a social phenomenon. *Instructional Science*, *14*(3–4), 381–438. https://doi.org/10.1007/BF00051829

Caron-Flinterman, J. F., Broerse, J. E. W., & Bunders, J. F. G. (2005). The experiential knowledge of patients: A new resource for biomedical research?. *Social Science & Medicine*, *60*(11), 2575–2584. https://doi.org/10.1016/j.socscimed.2004.11.023

Chappell, Z. (2023). In defence of the concept of mental illness. *Royal Institute of Philosophy Supplement*, *94*, 77–102. https://doi.org/10.1017/S1358246123000267

Conrad, P. (1992). Medicalization and social control. *Annual Review of Sociology*, *18*, 209–232. https://doi.org/10.1146/annurev.so.18.080192.001233

Cross, R., Davis, S., & O'Neil, I. (2017). *Health communication: Theoretical and critical perspectives*. Polity Press.

Davin, S. (2003). Healthy viewing: The reception of medical narratives. *Sociology of Health & Illness*, *25*(6), 662–679. https://doi.org/10.1111/1467-9566.00364

Deetz, S., & Mumby, D. K. (1990). Power, discourse, and the workplace: Reclaiming the critical tradition. *Annals of the International Communication Association*, *13*(1), 18–47. https://doi.org/10.1080/23808985.1990.11678743

Dumes, A. A. (2020). Lyme disease and the epistemic tensions of "medically unexplained illnesses". *Medical Anthropology*, *39*(6), 441–456. https://doi.org/10.1080/01459740.2019.1670175

Dutta, M. J. (2008). *Communicating health: A culture-centered approach*. Polity Press.

Dutta, M. J. (2010). The critical cultural turn in health communication: Reflexivity, solidarity, and praxis. *Health Communication*, *25*(6–7), 534–539. https://doi.org/10.1080/10410236.2010.497995

Dutton, W. H. (2009). The fifth estate emerging through the network of networks. *Prometheus*, *27*(1), 1–15. https://doi.org/10.1080/08109020802657453

Easterling, C. H. (2000). The social costs of treatment programs. *Journal of Religion and Health*, *39*(1), 43–49. https://doi.org/10.1023/A:1004690725027

Eden, D., & Bloor, J. (2010). Communication intelligence: Optimising healthcare communication in a digital age. *Journal of Communication in Healthcare*, *3*(2), 113–123. https://doi.org/10.1179/175380710X12813488575808

Eskola, K., & Puustinen, R. (1996). *Puhe, puukko, pilleri: Johdatusta terveyskeskuslääkärin työhön* [Speech, knife, pill: An introduction to the work of a health center doctor]. Duodecim.

Eyal, G. (2019). *The crisis of expertise*. Polity Press.

Foucault, M. (1994). *The birth of the clinic: An archaeology of medical perception*. Vintage Books. (Original work publihsed 1963)

Gadamer, H.-G. (1993). *Über die Verborgenheit der Gesundheit: Aufsätze und Vorträge* [On the enigma of health: Essays and lectures]. Suhrkamp.

Gadamer, H.-G. (1996). *The enigma of health: The art of healing in a scientific age*. Polity Press.

Groleau, D. (2011). Embodying "health citizenship" in health knowledge to fight health inequalities. *Revista Brasileira de Enfermagem*, *64*(5), 811–816. https://doi.org/10.1590/S0034-71672011000500002

Harjula, M. (2015). *Hoitoonpääsyn hierarkiat: Terveyskansalaisuus ja terveyspalvelut Suomessa 1900-luvulla* [Hierarchies of access to care: Health citizenship and health services in Finland in the 20th century]. Tampere University Press.

Helles, R. (2016). Communication types. In K. B. Jensen & R. T. Craig (Eds.), *The international encyclopedia of communication theory and philosophy*. Wiley. https://doi.org/10.1002/9781118766804.wbiect257

Ho, E. Y., Bylund, C. L., Van Weert, J. C. M., Basnyat, I., Bol, N., & Dean, M. (2023). *The international encyclopedia of health communication*. Wiley Blackwell.

Hofmann, B. (2001). Complexity of the concept of disease as shown through rival theoretical frameworks. *Theoretical Medicine and Bioethics*, *22*(3), 211–236. https://doi.org/10.1023/A:1011416302494

Hofmann, B. (2002). On the triad disease, illness and sickness. *The Journal of Medicine and Philosophy*, *27*(6), 651–673. https://doi.org/10.1076/jmep.27.6.651.13793

Hofmann, B. (2016). Disease, illness, and sickness. In M. Solomon, J. R. Simon, & H. Kincaid (Eds.), *The Routledge companion to philosophy of medicine* (pp. 16–26). Routledge.

ICIJ. (n.d.). *Implant files*. https://www.icij.org/investigations/implant-files/

Jauho, M., & Helén, I. (2023). Citizenship by vitality: Rethinking the concept of health citizenship. *Distinktion: Journal of Social Theory*, *24*(3), 467–487. https://doi.org/10.1080/1600910X.2022.2057561

Jensen, K. B., & Helles, R. (2011). The internet as a cultural forum: Implications for research. *New Media & Society*, *13*(4), 517–533. https://doi.org/10.1177/1461444810373531

Karlsen, M.-M. W., Holm, A., Kvande, M. E., Dreyer, P., Tate, J. A., Heyn, L. G., & Happ, M. B. (2023). Communication with mechanically ventilated patients in intensive care units: A concept analysis. *Journal of Advanced Nursing*, *79*(2), 563–580. https://doi.org/10.1111/jan.15501

Kleinman, A. (1988). *The illness narratives: Suffering, healing, and the human condition*. Basic Books.

Kreps, G. L. (2020). The value of health communication scholarship: New directions for health communication inquiry. *International Journal of Nursing Sciences*, *7*(S1), S4–S7. https://doi.org/10.1016/j.ijnss.2020.04.007

Kreps, G. L., Bonaguro, E. W., & Query Jr, J. L. (1998). The history and development of the field of health communication. In L. D. Jackson & B. K. Duffy (Eds.), *Health communication research: A guide to developments and directions* (pp. 1–15). Greenwood Press.

Laaksonen, M., Gould, R., & Liukko, J. (2018). Labor market position after a rejection of a disability pension application: A register-based cohort study. *Disability and Rehabilitation*, *40*(25), 3022–3029. https://doi.org/10.1080/09638288.2017.1367039

Lupton, D. (1993). The construction of patienthood in medical advertising. *International Journal of Social Determinants of Health and Health Services*, *23*(4), 805–819. https://doi.org/10.2190/FPDH-CXKD-RJH3-8REJ

Lupton, D. (1994). Toward the development of critical health communication praxis. *Health Communication*, *6*(1), 55–67. https://doi.org/10.1207/s15327027hc0601_4

Lupton, D. (1995). *The imperative of health: Public health and the regulated body*. SAGE Publications.

Lupton, D. (2003). *Medicine as culture: Illness, disease and the body in Western societies* (2nd ed.). SAGE Publications.

Marshall, T. H. (2009). Citizenship and social class. In J. Manza & M. Sauder (Eds.), *Inequality and society: Social science perspectives on social stratification* (pp. 148–154). W. W. Norton & Company.

Mazanderani, F., Noorani, T., Dudhwala, F., & Kamwendo, Z. T. (2020). Knowledge, evidence, expertise? The epistemics of experience in contemporary healthcare. *Evidence & Policy*, *16*(2), 267–284. https://doi.org/10.1332/174426420X15808912561112

McPhee, R. D., & Zaug, P. (2000). The communicative constitution of organization: A framework for explanation. *Electronic Journal of Communication*, *10*(1–2). https://www.cios.org/EJCPUBLIC/010/1/01017.html

Motamedi, M., Carter, S. M., & Degeling, C. (2023). Transvaginal mesh in Australia: An analysis of news media reporting from 1996 to 2021. *Health Expectations*, *26*(3), 1189–1201. https://doi.org/10.1111/hex.13734

Mumby, D. K. (2016). Organizations–made by communication, makers of communication. In K. B. Jensen & R. T. Craig (Eds.), *The international encyclopedia of communication theory and philosophy*. Wiley. https://doi.org/10.1002/9781118766804.wbiect131

Naukkarinen, J. (2004). Gadamer ja käytännöllinen lääketiede [Philosophy and practical medicine]. *Niin & Näin*, *3*(04), 119. https://netn.fi/artikkelit/gadamer-ja-kaytannollinen-laaketiede/

Neittaanmäki, P., & Kaasalainen, K. (2018). *SOTE-toimintojen tehostaminen IT:n avulla: kehittämispotentiaali ja toimenpideohjelma* [Improving the efficiency of social and health activities through IT – development potential and action plan]. Jyväskylän yliopisto.

Nettleton, S. (2006). "I just want permission to be ill": Towards a sociology of medically unexplained symptoms. *Social Science & Medicine*, *62*(5), 1167–1178. https://doi.org/10.1016/j.socscimed.2005.07.030

Noar, S. M., Barker, J., Bell, T., & Yzer, M. (2020). Does perceived message effectiveness predict the actual effectiveness of tobacco education messages? A systematic review and meta-analysis. *Health Communication*, *35*(2), 148–157. https://doi.org/10.1080/10410236.2018.1547675

Noar, S. M., Palmgreen, P., & Zimmerman, R. S. (2009). Reflections on evaluating health communication campaigns. *Communication Methods & Measures*, *3*(1–2), 105–114. https://doi.org/10.1080/19312450902809730

Parsons, T. (1951). Illness and the role of the physician: A sociological perspective. *American Journal of Orthopsychiatry*, *21*(3), 452–460. https://doi.org/10.1111/j.1939-0025.1951.tb00003.x

Piera-Jiménez, J., Carot-Sans, G., Ramiro-Pareta, M., Nogueras, M. M., Folguera-Profitós, J., Ródenas, P., Jiménez-Rueda, A., Navarro, T. D., Palacios,

J. A. M., Fajardo, J. C., Campillo, J. U., Vela, E., Monterde, D., Valero-Bover, D., Bonet, T., Tarrasó-Urios, G., Cantenys-Sabà, R., Fabregat-Fabregat, P., Oliveros, B. G.,. . . Pérez-Sust, P. (2024). A 25-Year retrospective of health IT infrastructure building: The example of the catalonia region. *Journal of Medical Internet Research*, *26*, e58933. https://doi.org/10.2196/58933

Pietilä, V. (2005). *On the highway of mass communication studies*. Hampton Press.

Prasad, A. J. (2022). Drapetomania: History of how psychiatry allowed itself to be abused by racists. *The Indian Practitioner*, *75*(2), 39–41. https://articles.theindianpractitioner.com/index.php/tip/article/view/1317

Putnam, L. L., Nicotera, A. M., & McPhee, R. (2009). Instruction communication constitutes organization. In L. L. Putnam & A. M. Nicotera (Eds.), *Building theories of organization: The constitutive role of communication* (pp. 1–20). Routledge.

Saborido, C., & García-Barranquero, P. (2022). Is aging a disease? The theoretical definition of aging in the light of the philosophy of medicine. *The Journal of Medicine and Philosophy: A Forum for Bioethics and Philosophy of Medicine*, *47*(6), 770–783. https://doi.org/10.1093/jmp/jhac030

Sadegh-Zadeh, K. (2000). Fuzzy health, illness, and disease: Polymorphic medical ontologies: Fashioning concepts of health and disease. *The Journal of Medicine and Philosophy: A Forum for Bioethics and Philosophy of Medicine*, *25*(5), 605–638. https://doi.org/10.1076/0360-5310(200010)25:5;1-W;FT605

Sarangi, S. (2018). Communicative expertise: The mutation of expertise and expert systems in contemporary professional practice. *Journal of Applied Linguistics and Professional Practice*, *13*(1–3), 371–392. https://doi.org/10.1558/japl.37507

Sendra, A. (2019). *Health communication processes in social media: Towards a transformative intervention on the information about chronic pain* [Doctoral dissertation, Universitat Rovira i Virgili]. Tesis Doctorals en Xarxa.

Sendra, A., Torkkola, S., & Govender, E. (2021). The breakthrough of digital health: Communication as the catalyst of the transformation of care [Editorial]. *Catalan Journal of Communication & Cultural Studies*, *13*(2), 169–178. https://doi.org/10.1386/cjcs_00047_2

Sendra, A., Torkkola, S., & Parviainen, J. (2023). Non-knowledge in medical practices: Approaching the uses of social media in healthcare from an epistemological perspective. *Journal of Digital Social Research*, *5*(1), 70–89. https://doi.org/10.33621/jdsr.v5i1.152

Sendra, A., Torkkola, S., & Parviainen, J. (2024). Astrazeneca vaccine controversies in the media: Theorizing about the mediatization of ignorance in the context of the COVID-19 vaccination Campaign. *Health Communication*, *39*(3), 541–551. https://doi.org/10.1080/10410236.2023.2171951

Showalter, E. (1998). *Hystories: Hysterical epidemics and modern culture*. Picador.

Snyder, L. B., Hamilton, M. A., Mitchell, E. W., Kiwanuka-Tondo, J., Fleming-Milici, F., & Proctor, D. (2004). A meta-analysis of the effect of mediated health communication campaigns on behavior change in the United States. *Journal of Health Communication*, *9*(sup1), 71–96. https://doi.org/10.1080/10810730490271548

Susser, M. (1990). Disease, illness, sickness; impairment, disability and handicap. *Psychological Medicine*, *20*(3), 471–473. https://doi.org/10.1017/S0033291700016974

Thomas, R. K. (2010). *Health communication*. Springer.

Torkkola, S. (2008). *Sairas juttu: Tutkimus terveysjournalismin teoriasta ja sanomalehden sairaalasta* [Sick story: Research on the theory of health journalism and the newspaper hospital]. Tampere University Press.

Torkkola, S. (2016). Multifaceted Health Communication. In V. Marinescu & B. Mitu (Eds.), *Health and the media: Essays on the effects of mass communication* (pp. 17–31). McFarland & Company, Inc.

Torkkola, S. (2018, June). *Healthcare communication in the era of digitalization* [Paper presentation]. International Association for Media and Communication Research (IAMCR) Conference 2018, Eugene (Oregon), USA.

Torkkola, S., Tyni, P., Parviainen, J., & Sendra, A. (2024). Terveydenhuollon muuttuvat viestintäkäytännöt: Kyselytutkimus terveydenhuollon asiantuntijoille sosiaalisen median mahdollisuuksista ja uhista potilastyössä [Changing practices in healthcare communication: A survey for healthcare experts about opportunities and threats of social media in patient care]. *Media & Viestintä*, *47*(4), 53–78. https://doi.org/10.23983/mv.130759

Twaddle, A. (1994). Disease, illness och sickness på nytt [Disease, illness and sickness again]. In B. Richt (Ed.), *Öppningar och farhågor. Fjorton humanister om hälsa, sjukdom och hälsofrämjande* (pp. 17–33). Linköpings universitet.

Twaddle, A., & Nordenfelt, L. (1994). *Disease, illness and sickness: Three central concepts in the theory of health*. Linköpings universitet.

Vaagan, R. W., Torkkola, S., Sendra, A., Farré, J., & Lovari, A. (2021). A critical analysis of the digitization of healthcare communication in the EU: A comparison of Italy, Finland, Norway, and Spain. *International Journal of Communication*, *15*, 1718–1740. https://ijoc.org/index.php/ijoc/article/view/15399

Viswanathan, K. (2008). Health communication. In W. Donsbach (Ed.), *The international encyclopedia of communication*. John Wiley & Sons. https://doi.org/10.1002/9781405186407.wbiech009

WHO. (1998, June 16). *Health promotion glossary*. https://www.who.int/publications/i/item/WHO-HPR-HEP−98.1

WHO. (2021, December 6). *Health promotion glossary of terms 2021*. https://www.who.int/publications/i/item/9789240038349

Wright, K. B., Sparks, L., & O'Hair, D. (2008). *Health communication in the 21st century*. Blackwell Publishing.

Wulff, H. R., Pedersen, S. A., & Rosenberg, R. (1990). *Philosophy of medicine: An introduction* (2nd ed.). Blackwell Scientific Publications.

Zola, I. K. (1972). Medicine as an institution of social control. *The Sociological Review*, *20*(4), 487–504. https://doi.org/10.1111/j.1467-954X.1972.tb00220.x

3 Digitalization of illness

From paternalism to empowerment

With the digital transformation of healthcare, there is one crucial question that remains to be answered in the context of patienthood: how has the experience of being ill from the perspective of the patient (i.e., illness) changed in the era of digitalization? For some, such as those living with chronic conditions, the digitalization of healthcare has opened the door to feeling less lonely while increasing the visibility of their illnesses (Sendra & Farré, 2020; Wright, 2016). As May (2006, p. 161, emphasis in original) reminds us in an editorial for *Chronic Illness*, "being ill *is* hard and heavy work" – thus, in a way, one could say that healthcare digitalization has improved the experience of being ill for those living with chronic conditions. However, the experience of being ill in the digital era has changed for all citizens, even for those who see themselves as healthy. In other words, as individuals, we are constantly exposed to a variety of information sources that might influence decision-making processes related to our health.

On this basis, social media has become one of the most common channels through which people obtain and discuss health knowledge. Regarding the acquisition of health knowledge, the COVID-19 crisis is one of the last examples of how these online platforms every day present us with contradictory information from multiple formal and informal sources, thus affecting our construction of health knowledge (López-Rico et al., 2020; Lovari, 2020). Concerning the distribution of health knowledge, in recent years individuals have been progressively using social media to talk about their experiences of being ill with others (see, e.g., Callard & Perego, 2021). These disembodied discussions democratize modern medicine, making us (as patient-citizens) feel more empowered (Lupton, 2014) to the point that healthcare professionals are sometimes left out of the online conversations around the experience of being ill (Karlsson et al., 2024; Sendra & Farré, 2020). As a result, power struggles between care receivers and care providers around the experience of being ill might eventually come to the surface (Benetoli et al., 2018), challenging the authoritarian one-way communication model commonly present in the provision and delivery of healthcare.

DOI: 10.4324/9781003519607-3

The case of social media, which is one of the latest and possibly most significant examples of virtual medicine, shows in a simple way how healthcare digitalization has brought both light and darkness to the experience of being ill. These effects, which one could argue are intrinsic to any digital transformation process, will guide the discussion related to the digitalization of illness and the changes around the experience of being ill. The chapter is divided as follows. First, we will discuss what it means to be ill from the perspective of the patient and why it is important to consider these experiences in healthcare. Second, we will outline how patients talked about illness before the digitalization of healthcare. Third, we will discuss how this digital transformation is changing the experience of being ill (and, by extension, patienthood). The final part of the chapter will deal with potential threats relating to the digitalization of illness before presenting the conclusion.

3.1 The experience of being ill from the perspective of the patient

Unlike disease, illness "has emotions and experience, such as anxiety, fear, pain, and suffering, as its basic phenomena" (Hofmann, 2016, p. 17). Thus, the focus of the experience of being ill is on the patient rather than on society (sickness) or the healthcare professional (disease). Based on subjectivity (Sendra et al., 2023), illness can provide us with knowledge that cannot be detected through evidence and/or is not institutionalized (Hofmann, 2016). Therefore, it is safe to assume that the experience of being ill from the perspective of the patient sometimes comprises knowledge that only the patients themselves can identify, thus highlighting its relevance for the practice of medicine. In most cases, the illness perspective coincides with those of society (sickness) and healthcare professionals (disease). However, controversies arise even when one of these perspectives misaligns with the others (Hofmann, 2016). Historically, this has been the case with conditions like multiple chemical sensitivity, chronic fatigue syndrome, and fibromyalgia (Alameda-Cuesta et al., 2021), where it can be challenging to obtain a leave of absence from responsibilities such as work, and there is still no test to objectively determine their presence in the patient's body. For people who live with these conditions, only the illness perspective is present.

To date, several studies have denominated the knowledge arising from the patient perspective as "experiential knowledge" (Borkman, 1976; Blume, 2017), and it includes information on both embodied (i.e., bodily symptoms) and disembodied experiences (e.g., cancelled appointments with the doctor) (Sendra et al., 2023). Likewise, knowledge arising from the patient perspective can come both from patients themselves and from those closest to them, like caregivers (Abel & Browner, 1998; Sendra et al., 2022). In combination with expert knowledge (i.e., the disease perspective), experiential knowledge provides a more nuanced understanding of the experience of being ill. In other words, the knowledge arising from the patient perspective "goes beyond the medical dimension, including elements that also affect the social sphere of these individuals" (Sendra et al., 2022, p. 114). The problem remains that not all doctors welcome experiential knowledge during the medical encounter, especially when this type of expertise has been generated with the support of resources such as social media (Sendra et al., 2023). When the experience of being ill is mostly measured through evidence-based practices, the doctor is inevitably placed in a position of authority over the patient, thus creating what Carel and Kidd (2017) denote as "knowledge asymmetries". In fact, an example of knowledge asymmetry consists of "privileging the knowledge derived from medical training and theory, rather than that potentially rooted in patient experience" (Carel & Kidd, 2017, p. 336).

The way in which health knowledge is constructed in the medical encounter was recently studied by Magnussen et al. (2024). Through an analysis of interview data with healthcare professionals and patients living with hand osteoarthritis and evidence from multiple observations of their medical encounters, Magnussen et al. identified up to four different positions from which health knowledge is constructed between patients and healthcare professionals (Magnussen et al., 2024). These positions range from the more hierarchical to the more participatory, where the experiential knowledge leads the consultation. Theoretically, at least two of these positions ("from patients as knowers in the chronic healthcare dialogue, from health professionals and patients constructing knowledge together") recognize the importance of the experience of being ill from the perspective of the patient (Magnussen et al., 2024, Results section, para. 1). Nevertheless, the study also concludes that the construction of health knowledge from the identified positions seems to depend on "how strongly they are voiced" (Magnussen et al., 2024, Discussion section, para. 1). While the medical encounter is now much more participatory than it used to be (Killbride & Joffe, 2018; Timmermans, 2020), the reality is that experiential knowledge is still not fully appreciated as knowledge with the capacity to complement expert knowledge, especially in cases where only the illness perspective is present (Carel & Kidd, 2017).

In this context, narrative medicine (Charon, 2001a) is one of the few approaches to healthcare – if not the only one – that puts the experience of being ill from the perspective of the patient at the centre of the medical practice. In fact, narrative medicine is rooted in the idea that "scientifically competent medicine alone cannot help a patient grapple with the loss of health or find meaning in suffering" (Charon, 2001b, p. 1897). In other words, (objective) evidence is not enough to manage the experience of being ill from the perspective of the patient. Arguments in favour of structuring the medical practice around illness were already published in earlier studies (see, e.g., Frank, 1995; Hydén, 1997; Kleinman, 1988). However, it was Charon (2001a, p. 83) who first conceptualized narrative medicine as "medicine practiced with the narrative competence to recognize, interpret, and be moved to action by the predicaments of others".

At the intersection between the humanities and medicine, the challenge of this type of medical practice is for healthcare professionals to receive the necessary training to interpret the narratives of illness told by patients (Charon, 2006). Another obstacle is the variety of methods and rigour applied to exercise narrative medicine (Charon, 2021). The importance of narratives for describing the experience of being ill from the perspective of the patient is described in detail in the next section.

3.2 Narratives to construct and make sense of the experience of being ill

In simple terms, the experience of being ill is a disruption of what is known as normality in the life of an individual. This irregularity, which might vary in seriousness depending on the condition experienced, always involves a disturbance of how things usually are, even when the disruption is only temporary (Hydén, 1997). For example, a person is forced to reduce the intensity of their training when doing exercise (disembodied experience) because they start experiencing pain in the body that was not there before (embodied experience). To explain these changes and generate experiential knowledge, patients rely on storytelling, using narratives to understand and make sense of their new reality (Frank, 1995). In fact, previous studies show how narratives play a fundamental role in the construction of experiential knowledge when it comes to chronic illnesses (Hydén, 1997; Sendra et al., 2022). Moreover, "narratives not only articulate suffering but also give the sufferer a voice for articulating the illness experience apart from how illnesses are conceived and represented by biomedicine" (Hydén, 1997, p. 51). In other words, narratives not only seem to be inherent to the experience of being ill from the perspective of the patient, but they also help these individuals to talk about their conditions on their own terms.

The study of narratives in the context of illness started to gain relevance in the late 1980s and early 1990s (Kleinman, 1988). One of the first authors to provide a framework for analysing illness narratives was Arthur W. Frank (1995), who categorized illness narratives into restitution (where the patient expects a return to normality after going through the illness), chaos (where the illness becomes the new normality for the patient), and quest (where the illness has a purpose for the patient to learn). Later, Hydén (1997) proposed classifying illness narratives into illness as narrative (where the illness is constructed via the narrative), narrative about illness (where information regarding the illness is provided through the narrative), and narrative as illness (where an ill narrative defines the illness). While Frank's (1995) categories are based on the illness trajectory of the patient, Hydén's (1997, p. 54) follow the "ways in which narrator, illness and narrative may be interrelated". Another typology can be found in the work of Bury (2001), who categorized illness narratives into contingent narratives (where the narrative discusses impressions of the origins of illness and its consequences for patients), moral narratives (where the narrative deals with the impacts of illness on the social dimension of patients), and core narratives (where the narrative discloses how the experience of being ill is influenced by the cultural settings of the patient). Being closer to Frank's (1995) rather than Hydén's (1997) research, the categorization offered by Bury (2001, p. 281) is based on "the links between body, self and society".

Collectively, these studies outline the multiple ways in which patients construct and make sense of their experiences of being ill, while providing us with an extensive framework to interpret illness narratives in terms of both content (Bury, 2001; Frank, 1995) and format (Hydén, 1997). Likewise, they also show how significant (and influential) social factors are in describing illness, which brings us to our next point. The construction of the experience of being ill does not happen in a vacuum; it is shaped by what Klawiter (2004, p. 851) describes as disease regimes, which "are comprised of the institutionalised practices, authoritative discourses, social relations, collective identities, emotional vocabularies, visual images, public policies and regulatory actions through which diseases are socially constituted and experienced". Therefore, while narratives provide power to the patient to talk about illness, they still need to share their stories within a disease regime (i.e., a social structure) where the institutionalized practice is to consider illness as inferior in comparison to disease (Kleinman, 1988). This superiority of the healthcare professionals' perspective is already established during their education, where the acquisition of competence – rooted in basic research – trumps caring attitudes as their training advances (Good & Good, 1993). In turn, the more competence healthcare professionals acquire, the greater is the gap created between the patient and healthcare professional, as "[t]he specialized knowledge of the professional creates the basis for prestige and social distance between the expert and the client [patient]" (Turner, 1987, p. 135).

Prior to the era of digitalization, the supremacy of disease tended to silence illness (Frank, 1995). Patients had little room for exercising their patienthood from the perspective of illness beyond their network of strong ties (Sendra et al., 2023). Moreover, not only were disease discourses imposed in their encounters with healthcare professionals, but the disease regime under which the experience of being ill was managed would often not consider any resolution other than recovery (Frank, 1995). Even though patients had the means (i.e., storytelling) to discuss illness, their voices tended to be silenced when expressed outside the private sphere (Kleinman, 1988). As previously stated, recent evidence indicates that contemporary medical practices still sometimes work under this type of disease regime (Magnussen et al., 2024). However, thanks to the digital era, healthcare professionals have had to adopt more participatory practices (Timmermans, 2020), opening new avenues for patients to talk about the experience of being ill from their perspective. As Erikainen et al. (2019, Datafication and the construction of community section, para. 2) argue, "digital and social media have innovated patient options for interacting, generating networks, forming identities and communities, and mobilising in unprecedented ways". These and other changes will be discussed thoroughly in the following section.

3.3 Digitalizing the experience of being ill

As we saw in the previous section, illness narratives and experiential knowledge existed long before the digitalization of healthcare communication. However, digitalization has brought significant changes to the experience of being ill from the perspective of the patient (Table 3.1). Online communities and the information exchanged in them are now part of the unlimited information sources through which patients construct experiential knowledge (Karlsson et al., 2024). Thus, instead of disregarding and downplaying what happens inside them (Sendra et al., 2023), online communities should be embraced as spaces where illness and the experience of being ill are constructed and documented in ways that can improve both the organization and delivery of healthcare. Stage et al. (2024, p. 53) remind us that peer-led online communities

> not only serve as spaces for building bodily expertise – about e.g. what kind of everyday interventions might alleviate various conditions or illnesses – but also for building systemic expertise as a shared resource based on the broader collective's experiences with healthcare institutions and professionals.

The following illustrates how the digitalization of illness is facilitating patient empowerment (Sosnowy, 2014) from different perspectives, focusing on describing how participating in online communities is changing the exercise of patienthood.

One of the most documented changes for patients with regard to the digitalization of illness is the increased access to social support, especially of the informational and emotional kind. Early examples of research into the perceived

Table 3.1 Changes to the experience of being ill from the perspective of the care receiver brought by digitalization

Changes	*References*
Online communities . . .	
. . .increase access to social support	Ressler et al. (2012), Sosnowy (2014), Gonzalez-Polledo (2016), Sendra and Farré (2020)
. . .enable the networked co-construction of experiential knowledge	Gonzalez-Polledo and Tarr (2016), Sendra et al. (2023), Cao and Wang (2024)
. . .have a role in addressing health controversies	Jackson (2023)
. . .help patients share non-institutionalized narratives, thus contributing to the continuity of care	Sendra and Farré (2020), Stage et al. (2024)
. . .promote multimodal expressions of the experience of being ill	Gonzalez-Polledo and Tarr (2016), Cao and Wang (2024)

benefits of participating in online communities include, to name a few, the work of Ressler et al. (2012), Sosnowy (2014), Gonzalez-Polledo (2016), and Sendra and Farré (2020). A common trait in these studies is that they all deal with non-acute conditions, such as chronic pain. This shows how healthcare delivery models have historically neglected some of the needs of these patients (OECD/EU, 2022), forcing them to meet their desires elsewhere – like in online communities. In fact, "limited access to adequate support within traditional social network(s)" (Wright, 2016, p. 68) is one of the indicators that prompt patients to take part in, for example, a Facebook group centred on one's condition. Participating in these online communities makes patients feel less isolated (Gonzalez-Polledo, 2016; Ressler et al., 2012; Sendra & Farré, 2020) and more informed about their illnesses (Sosnowy, 2014). Moreover, patients perceive that they are regaining control over their own lives by helping others (Ressler et al., 2012) and having "the ability and option to influence their treatment" (Sosnowy, 2014, p. 322).

With this increased access to information, patients are also co-constructing knowledge around their experiences of being ill in a different way. As we discussed previously in this chapter, illness narratives were present in healthcare long before the digital era (Williams, 1984; Hydén, 1997). However, what has changed with digitalization is how these narratives are being generated. For example, patients are now able to discuss their symptoms with other peers beyond the shadow of paternalism imposed by evidence-based medicine, forming networked narratives that reveal (previously) undiscovered aspects of their conditions (Cao & Wang, 2024; Gonzalez-Polledo & Tarr, 2016; Sendra et al., 2023). These stories include knowledge on both bodily expertise that might not be easily identified through objective measurements and the patients' experiences with healthcare (Sendra et al., 2023; Stage et al., 2024) – knowledge that can later be used by different groups (if accessed) to improve services for patients (see, e.g., Sendra et al., 2022). While the nature of the illness narratives shared online remains individual (Cao & Wang, 2024), the power of these stories rests in their collective interpretation, which in the case of long COVID "provided a rich description of the diverse manifestations of a grave new illness, a shared account of rejection by the healthcare system, and a powerful call for action to fix the broken story" (Rushforth et al., 2021, Summary of main findings section, para. 1).

An increasing body of evidence supports the fact that long COVID is the first illness defined through social media, thanks to the experiential knowledge shared by patients in different online communities dedicated to the condition (Callard & Perego, 2021; Rushforth et al., 2021). However, it should be noted that not everyone participates in online communities in the same way. For example, Maslen and Lupton (2019) have explored how Australian women used Facebook for constructing health knowledge to reveal three different modes of engagement: observation (the most common), appropriating expertise (usually built over time), and sharing personal experiences. In addition to having a more active or passive role, a recent study by Karlsson et al. (2024) found that patients seem to participate more in online communities just after being diagnosed. In that moment, the knowledge available in online communities "functions as support and a primary source of knowledge alongside the medical expertise until they [the patients] render themselves experienced enough to withdraw to rely mostly on their own experiential knowledge" (Karlsson et al., 2024, p. 13). Against this background, it might be that patients with long COVID were quickly successful in their activism because the onset of the symptoms was experienced at the same time by thousands of individuals, prompting them to simultaneously take part in online communities and thus constructing long COVID through shared experiences.

Unfortunately, this "joint" temporality concerning the onset of long COVID is not shared with other illnesses that have been trying to claim recognition for decades (Blease et al., 2017). In this context, the case of long COVID is also significant because it shows the potential of online communities with regard to addressing health controversies (Jackson, 2023). In contrast to (traditional) news media, the focus in online communities is on the individual frames of an illness, thus opening an avenue to discuss the experience of being ill beyond macro socio-economic perspectives that often overlook personal suffering (Cao & Wang, 2024). In other words, thanks to their practices of sharing personal experiences in spaces like social media, patients managed to "deinstitutionalize" (Jackson, 2023) the idea, further distributed (i.e., mediatized) by news media, that the SARS-CoV-2 infection only caused short-term symptoms. From this perspective, online communities are not only spaces to find comfort and improve patients' well-being but also an opportunity to "bring something profoundly different to the health communication environment. Under the right circumstances, they can enter science places and advance scientific positions of their own" (Jackson, 2023, p. 61). While this collective agency also existed before the digitalization of illness (e.g., through patient organizations), the characteristics of online communities enhanced the capacity of patients to act on their condition.

Likewise, illness narratives shared in online communities also help patients "fight against the status quo" (Sendra & Farré, 2020, p. 50). As previously discussed, what often prevails in patient–doctor relationships under the framework of paternalism and institutionalization is a narrative of recovery, where the experience of being ill is repeatedly managed with the objective of (full) restoration (Frank, 1995). However, several lines of evidence suggest that the experience of being ill is not always of this nature, especially for patients living with chronic conditions (Kleinman, 1988; Rushforth et al., 2021; Sendra & Farré, 2020). Sometimes, this objective of restoration simply means that patients reach a point of stability while waiting for the next flare up (i.e., worsening of symptoms) to manifest itself. In contrast to the typical encounter between patients and healthcare professionals, patients in online communities decide how to share their experiences with peers (in what Sendra & Farré,

2020, call the "reenactment phase"), thus opening an avenue for narratives not based on recovery to be at the forefront of the experience of being ill. When processed collectively, narratives shared in online communities are also used by patients to fill the gaps in their healthcare management, a process that Stage et al. (2024) denominated "systemic mending". In this context, systemic mending is defined as "patient-driven attempts to collectively gather and share information with peers that increase individual abilities to effectively navigate the healthcare system" (Stage et al., 2024, p. 51).

In addition to talking about the experience of being ill beyond the framework of restitution, online communities provide the opportunity to share experiential knowledge around illnesses in formats other than the spoken word, such as texts and images. In a study about chronic pain expressions on social media, Gonzalez-Polledo and Tarr (2016) found that images are widely used by patients to talk about the experience of being ill. Although their interpretation is not always clear, the authors suggest that images help these individuals evoke and make chronic pain visible while highlighting what it means to be ill. Conversely, Cao and Wang (2024) found that patients now seem to rely more on textual expressions to talk about the experience of being ill. To justify this change of format, the authors argue "that textual descriptions allow for a more imaginative portrayal of illness, while visual images often struggle with the nuanced dimensions of suffering, failing to capture internal and emotional pain aspects" (Cao &Wang, 2024, The expansion of social media logic in illness narrative section, para. 3). It should be noted that, while the analysis of Gonzalez-Polledo and Tarr (2016) focuses on image-based social media platforms such as Flickr and Tumblr, the study by Cao and Wang (2024) is centred on the instant-messaging app WeChat, which might explain the preference for text instead of images among their findings. In any case, what both studies show is that online communities allow for multimodal expressions of experiential knowledge that, when analysed together, can expand our understanding of the experience of being ill (Gonzalez-Polledo & Tarr, 2016).

All these significant changes to the experience of being ill from the perspective of the patient brought by digitalization (Table 3.1) have altered the interactions between the care provider and the care receiver. From the perspective of medicine, a doctor meets a more informed patient whose knowledge is not based only on the experience of being ill but also on medical information that previously was not available to laypeople (see, e.g., Lupton, 2018; Sendra et al., 2024). Patients use medical information in their own ways as well, which at times can be contradictory to the medical information provided by healthcare professionals. For example, on the Finnish online service Suomi24 (Finland24) there is a discussion group where the participants share their experience of medication, such as the adverse reactions and effects of medication (Torkkola, 2016a, 2016b). In this context, there was a long discussion chain for years focusing on a strong painkiller, Tramal, and its use to cure depression (Torkkola, 2016a, 2016b). The information found on social media and the Internet utilized by patients is often information that the doctor and other healthcare professionals do not know or accept (Sendra et al., 2023). In extreme situations, information of this kind can cause a conflict between the care provider and the care receiver (Torkkola et al., 2024). Thus, expertise, constructed through communication between the care provider and the care receiver, can progress to mutual understanding and care, but it can also be a source of conflict. These changes in the relationship between the care provider and the care receiver need more attention from healthcare professionals and healthcare organizations more broadly.

3.4 Risks associated with the digitalization of illness

The previous section has shown how the digitalization of illness has changed patienthood for the better. In the digital era, the experience of being ill from the perspective of the patient is more noticeable (see Callard & Perego, 2021), and health-related decision-making processes are more balanced thanks to patients' increased access to information sources and personal options for quantifying the body, such as wearables that provide detailed data on heart and/or respiratory rates. As a result, medicine is now more democratic, allowing patients to challenge and deconstruct disease regimes anchored in old and authoritarian practices. Nevertheless, the digitalization of illness has also entailed the rise of a variety of challenges both for the patient and the healthcare professional, which in the long run may represent a risk to public health. As Timmermans (2020, p. 269) argues, "[i]t is clear, though, that engaged patienthood also has drawbacks, specifically when engagement does not benefit a patient's health and physicians relent under patient pressure". For example, what happens when the construction of experiential knowledge is based on dis- and misinformation, as it transpired – especially in terms of vaccine hesitancy; see Khullar (2022) or Sendra et al. (2024) – during the COVID-19 pandemic? In fact, vaccines have traditionally been one of the areas most affected by dis- and misinformation (Encinillas-García & Martín-Sabarís, 2023). The discussion below is intended to reflect on these difficulties while highlighting potential ways to address them.

With the digitalization of illness, patients now have the option to diagnose themselves using resources like social media, where they discuss their symptoms with other peers without the intervention of healthcare professionals. From this perspective, one could say that illness narratives are inevitably influenced by the logic of the media. According to recent research (Sendra et al., 2024), the risk for this process of biomediatization (Briggs & Hallin, 2016) is to reach a point of no return, where the narratives surrounding a condition are completely controlled by the logic of the media. Likewise, disembodied social media discussions in which laypeople oversee their own narratives can differ quite significantly from disembodied mass media discussions. As Lee (2023, p. 487) and others (Sola-Pueyo, 2022) have shown, "health knowledge does not flow linearly from scientists to the [. . .] public. Journalists select the information that lay people need to know and present collected materials as medical facts". Consequently, biomediatization processes may lead to contrasting narratives of the same phenomenon. If patienthood now involves collectively engaging in online disembodied discussions of illness that avoid the mass media, then there is a need to further understand the social and cultural practices related to this. In this context, Van Dijck and Alinejad (2020) call for a networked model of science communication when publicly discussing illness in which patienthood and its related disembodied social media discussions are included in the process of healthcare communication.

The rhetoric of empowerment arising from the digitalization of illness also hides a dark side rooted in the concept of (health) responsibilization (Erikainen et al., 2019; Farré-Coma & Sendra-Toset, 2021), which translates to the idea that patients – at the individual level – end up being primarily responsible for their state of health. The management of the COVID-19 pandemic is probably one of the latest examples of this problematic, where preventing infections heavily relied on the individual behaviours of citizens, such as wearing masks (Sendra et al., 2024). This transfer of responsibilities from healthcare professionals to patients is born from the neoliberal and individualistic logic of contemporary societies, where "[i]llness comes to be seen as an outward sign of neglect of one's corporeal self – a condition considered as shameful, dirty or irresponsible" (Brown & Baker, 2012, p. 28). To be better responsible for their state of health in the digital era, patients are expected to self-manage their conditions with the support of digital technologies (Varey et al., 2021). In addition to generating new forms of surveillance (Lupton, 2016, 2022), putting too heavy a focus on the individual overlooks the role of the social determinants in the management of a condition (Varey et al., 2021). As Erikainen et al. (2019, Commercialising and consuming health section, para. 5) remind us, "taking greater responsibility for one's own health can easily translate into increased expectations or obligations to maintain and promote personal health", and not all patients might have the means (or the willingness; see, e.g., Sosnowy, 2014) to meet them.

This idea of responsibilization is also reflected in the narratives around the experiences of being ill that patients share through online platforms like social media. In a recent study on Instagram and depression, Schaller et al. (2023) examined the effects of responsibility frames in social media illness narratives on the public discourse surrounding this condition. Particularly, the authors analysed the influence of three different frames, including individual (where the responsibility for a condition falls on the person who suffers from it), social (where the responsibility for a condition depends on the social network of the sufferer), and combination (where responsibility for a condition is a combination of both individual and social frames). For example, the authors found that when a narrative is structured around individual frames, the stigmatization towards depression (including self-stigmatization) might increase, thus having negative consequences for public health (e.g., isolation). In turn, when a narrative is structured around social frames, the stigmatization towards depression has the potential to decrease, thus contributing to increasing the social acceptance of the condition. Altogether, the results of the study "demonstrate that emphasizing different aspects of responsibility in Instagram posts significantly shapes the recipients' opinion about who is and who is not to blame for depression" (Schaller et al., 2023, p. 762). Therefore, patients not only run the risk of being solely responsible for managing their conditions in the digital era but also of blaming themselves for having become ill due to the public discourse surrounding their conditions, even to the point that the pressure experienced could become unbearable (Farré-Coma & Sendra-Toset, 2021).

In this context, the problem is not that patients were not responsible for their conditions in the past, but that they trusted in the information sources at their disposal, which were mainly healthcare professionals. If patients were lucky enough to live in an area with support groups and associations related to their condition, they could also incorporate experiential knowledge from other patients into their experiences of being ill. Rather, the issue is that patients now continue to be responsible for their conditions but with exponentially increased access to information sources that might generate confusion (Rodríguez-González, 2023) and cannot always be trusted, as they might be based on misinformation (Rodgers & Massac, 2020). Tackling misleading and false information is no easy task due to the nature of the misinformation itself. In health contexts, Krishna and Thompson (2021, p. 325) describe misinformation "as acceptance of false or (scientifically) inaccurate data as useful (a) despite exposure to (scientifically) accurate data, (b) in the absence of accurate data or messages to the contrary, or/and (c) within historical or contextual legacies". Given this complexity, the literature on misleading and false information has proposed several solutions to counteract misinformation related to health. For example, some studies suggest increased digital health literacy and media literacy for both patients and healthcare professionals (Lovari, 2020; Sendra et al., 2023). Other research advocates for multiple open communication channels from authorities, particularly during a health crisis (Lopes et al., 2023; Rodgers & Massac, 2020). Open communication channels from authorities (e.g., a Facebook page from a primary healthcare centre) are not only a way to counteract misinformation but also a fruitful method for promoting health education (Rodríguez-González, 2021). Meanwhile, Memenga et al. (2022) provide evidence that debunking strategies could be an effective way to tackle misleading and false information in health contexts, as previously suggested also by Dhawan et al. (2021). Regardless of the approach followed, this increasing amount of literature shows how critical it is to counteract misinformation related to health, not only to prevent a new infodemic (Lovari, 2020) but also to address a growing epidemic (Krishna & Thompson, 2021; Rodgers & Massac, 2020).

Lastly, the experience of being ill from the perspective of the patient is also subjected through digitalization to what Lupton (2014, p. 864) terms "the digital patient experience economy", "in which patients' experiences of illness and medical treatments and their opinions on health care as they are uploaded to online platforms have become valorised, and in some contexts, monetised". Particularly, illness narratives have biographical value (Mazanderani et al., 2013), where the act of sharing the experience of being ill is seen by patients as something valuable both to help others and oneself – to the point that, in some cases, illness narratives might end up generating a profit (e.g., through advertising). In this context, the biographical value of illness narratives in the digital era is exploited by individuals and companies alike (Lupton, 2014; Mazanderani et al., 2013), where the latter usually offer their services free of charge, "seeking to use the data collected for commercial reasons" (Lupton, 2014, p. 862). A recent study by Eriksson (2023) also argues that commodification, anchored in the logic of the market, can influence how illness narratives are constituted, thus losing in the process what made these stories unique in the first place. Rather than providing experiential knowledge useful for improving the organization and delivery of healthcare, the experiences of being ill from the perspective of the patient could materialize into a narrative that accommodates the existing institutionalized practices of old disease regimes. To minimize the effects of commodification, Eriksson (2023) concludes that healthcare professionals should engage in processes of self-reflection when exercising participatory medical practices.

In telemedicine and e-health, the lack of face-to-face interaction between the care receiver and the care provider has been seen as problematic because it can affect not only the specific treatment but also the diagnosis and decision-making process for the treatment, including in ways that are not yet understood (see, e.g., Lupton & Maslen, 2017; Matusitz & Breen, 2007; Parviainen & Rantala, 2022). If healthcare organizations do not pay attention to how communication has changed through digitalization and do not further educate healthcare professionals to adapt to virtual interactions with more empowered patients, trust in healthcare professionals and overall evidence-based medicine may be weakened (see Chapter 4, which focuses on medical disease, for a discussion of these challenges).

3.5 The consolidation of participatory patienthood

The aim of the present chapter was to explore in what ways the digital era has transformed illness. To do this, we drew on previous studies conducted by us and other researchers on the construction of health knowledge, the use of social media and other digital platforms for health-related purposes, and the medical encounters between patients and healthcare professionals. The most obvious finding to emerge from the discussion presented above is that patienthood is indeed now more participatory (Sosnowy, 2014), where individuals have more agency to voice their conditions from the perspective of illness both within and outside the medical encounter, thus challenging paternalistic disease regimes and advocating for the improvement of the organization and delivery of healthcare. However, it should be noted that participatory patienthood "simultaneously offers opportunities for patients to gain medical knowledge and resist medical patriarchy, as well as compounds expectations placed upon patients to assume greater responsibility for managing their care" (Sosnowy, 2014, p. 316). In neoliberal societies, patient empowerment can easily translate into unpaid, often unwanted labour resulting from expectations of responsibility (Lupton, 2022; Sosnowy, 2014), which in turn might result in more illness for patients due to the perceived pressures they experience to fulfil their role. For this reason, Varey et al. (2021, Discussion section, para. 2) propose a focus on the co-management (rather than self-management) of healthcare, where "patients, family carers and HCPs [healthcare professionals] adopt active roles in the management of patient healthcare", thus sharing the responsibility. Others (see, e.g., Grosjean et al., 2021) take this approach one step further and involve the patient in the design of the digital technologies that these individuals will later use to co-manage their condition.

In the era of digitalization, the concept of the patient as we knew it – i.e., as someone always "expected to comply" (Killbride & Joffe, 2018, p. 1973) with the decisions made by healthcare professionals on their behalf – does not stand true anymore. Instead, patienthood involves engaging in a series of actions that enrich the patient's knowledge and reduce dependence on healthcare professionals, opening an avenue for exercising less biased and more balanced medical practices. In doing so, patients generate communication practices driven by illness (i.e., based on their experiences), going one step further from patient-centred communication practices, where the experience of being ill from the perspective of the healthcare professional (i.e., disease) remains central to the provision and delivery of healthcare. However, this new understanding of the concept of the patient needs to be critically analysed in a systematic way (Lupton, 2022). As we have seen in this chapter, the reconstruction of patienthood risks falling into new versions of old disease regimes that simply reproduce existing patterns, but in a different way. Likewise, the digitalization of illness, under which this reconstructed patienthood operates, has affected healthcare communication at all levels: between patients and institutions (e.g., the co-production of science communication), between patients and care providers (e.g., the co-construction of health knowledge), and between patients themselves (e.g., enhanced activism, the capacity to generate scientific research). In this context, greater efforts are needed to keep up with these transformations, starting with the development of educational interventions (Francés-Tecles & Camaño-Puig, 2024; Mather & Cummings, 2019) that provide healthcare professionals with the necessary communicative expertise to better consider the experiences of being ill from the perspective of the patient in their medical practices.

Under the digitalization of healthcare communication, patienthood is a result of the collision between the expertise of the patient (experiential knowledge) and the expertise of the healthcare professional (expert knowledge), reconfiguring the social structures in which health knowledge is generated and providing the experience of being ill from the perspective of the patient (i.e., illness) a more relevant role in the communication processes of healthcare throughout the whole organization. Resulting from this reconstructed patienthood, the relationship between the patient and the experience of being ill from the perspective of the healthcare professional (i.e., disease) also becomes altered, where the epistemology of expert knowledge in modern medicine increasingly goes from biomedicine to virtual medicine. The consequences of this change for both patienthood and contemporary medical practices are discussed thoroughly in the rest of the book (see Chapter 4).

References

Abel, E. K., & Browner, C. H. (1998). Selective compliance with biomedical authority and the uses of experiential knowledge. In M. Lock & P. A. Kaufert (Eds.), *Pragmatic women and body politics* (pp. 310–326). Cambridge University Press.

Alameda-Cuesta, A., Pazos-Garciandía, A., Oter-Quintana, C., Losa-Iglesias, M. E. (2021). Fibromyalgia, chronic fatigue syndrome, and multiple chemical sensitivity: Illness experiences. *Clinical Nursing Research*, *30*(1), 32–41. https://doi.org/10.1177/1054773819838679

Benetoli, A., Chen, T. F., & Aslani, P. (2018). How patients' use of social media impacts their interactions with healthcare professionals. *Patient Education and Counseling*, *101*(3), 439–444. https://doi.org/10.1016/j.pec.2017.08.015

Blease, C., Carel, H., & Geraghty, K. (2017). Epistemic injustice in healthcare encounters: Evidence from chronic fatigue syndrome. *Journal of Medical Ethics*, *43*(8), 549–557. https://doi.org/10.1136/medethics-2016-103691

Blume, S. (2017). In search of experiential knowledge. *Innovation: The European Journal of Social Science Research*, *30*(1), 91–103. https://doi.org/10.1080/13511610.2016.1210505

Borkman, T. (1976). Experiential knowledge: A new concept for the analysis of self-help groups. *Social Service Review*, *50*(3), 445–456. https://doi.org/10.1086/643401

Briggs, C. L., & Hallin, D. C. (2016). *Making health public: How news coverage is remaking media, medicine, and contemporary life*. Routledge.

Brown, B. J., & Baker, S. (2012). *Responsible citizens: Individuals, health and policy under neoliberalism*. Anthem Press.

Bury, M. (2001). Illness narratives: Fact or fiction?. *Sociology of Health & Illness*, *23*(3), 263–285. https://doi.org/10.1111/1467-9566.00252

Callard, F., & Perego, E. (2021). How and why patients made long Covid. *Social Science & Medicine*, *268*, 113426. https://doi.org/10.1016/j.socscimed.2020.113426

Cao, B., & Wang, L. (2024). When epidemic outbreaks meet social media: Collective illness narratives on WeChat during COVID-19 Omicron infection in

China. *Health Communication*, *39*(11), 2211–2224. https://doi.org/10.1080/10410236.2023.2259695

Carel, H., & Kidd, I. J. (2017). Epistemic injustice in medicine and healthcare. In I. J. Kidd, J. Medina, & G. Pohlhaus Jr (Eds.), *The Routledge handbook of epistemic injustice* (pp. 336–346). Routledge.

Charon, R. (2001a). Narrative medicine: Form, function, and ethics. *Annals of Internal Medicine*, *134*(1), 83–87. https://www.acpjournals.org/doi/10.7326/0003-4819-134-1-200101020-00024

Charon, R. (2001b). Narrative medicine: A model for empathy, reflection, profession, and trust. *JAMA*, *286*(15), 1897–1902. https://doi.org/10.1001/jama.286.15.1897

Charon, R. (2006). *Narrative medicine: Honoring the stories of illness*. Oxford University Press.

Charon, R. (2021). Narrative medicine. In P. Crawford & P. Kadetz (Eds.), *Palgrave encyclopedia of the health humanities*. Palgrave Macmillan Cham. https://doi.org/10.1007/978-3-030-26825-1_36-1

Dhawan, D., Bekalu, M., Pinnamaneni, R., McCloud, R., & Viswanath, K. (2021). COVID-19 news and misinformation: Do they matter for public health prevention?. *Journal of Health Communication*, *26*(11), 799–808. https://doi.org/10.1080/10810730.2021.2010841

Encinillas-García, M., & Martín-Sabarís, R. M. (2023). Desinformación y salud en la era PRECOVID: Una revisión sistemática [Misinformation and health in the PRECOVID era: A systematic review]. *Revista de Comunicación y Salud*, *13*, 1–15. https://doi.org/10.35669/rcys.2023.13.e312

Erikainen, S., Pickersgill, M., Cunningham-Burley, S., & Chan, S. (2019). Patienthood and participation in the digital era. *Digital Health*, 5. https://doi.org/10.1177/2055207619845546

Eriksson, E. (2023). A market of lived experience – User involvement and the commodification of personal experiences of mental illness. *International Journal of Environmental Research and Public Health*, *20*(14), 6427. https://doi.org/10.3390/ijerph20146427

Farré-Coma, J., & Sendra-Toset, A. (2021). El giro hacia la centralidad transformadora del paciente en la salud digital: dilemas y retos [The turn towards the transforming centrality of the patient in digital health: Dilemmas and challenges]. In J. L. Terrón, C. Peñafiel, D. Catalán, & M. R. Rodríguez (Eds.), *Comunicación y promoción de la salud en la era digital* (pp. 17–33). Dykinson.

Francés-Tecles, E., & Camaño-Puig, R. (2024). Experiencia y percepción de las enfermeras respecto del proceso de comunicación con los pacientes [Experience and perceptions of nurses regarding the communication process with patients]. *Revista de Comunicación y Salud*, *14*, 1–15. https://doi.org/10.35669/rcys.2024.14.e342

Frank, A. W. (1995). *The wounded storyteller: Body, illness, and ethics*. The University of Chicago Press.

Gonzalez-Polledo, E. (2016). Chronic media worlds: Social media and the problem of pain communication on Tumblr. *Social Media + Society*, *2*(1), 1–11. https://doi.org/10.1177/2056305116628887

Gonzalez-Polledo, E., & Tarr, J. (2016). The thing about pain: The remaking of illness narratives in chronic pain expressions on social media. *New Media & Society*, *18*(8), 1455–1472. https://doi.org/10.1177/1461444814560126

Good, B. J., & Good, M. D. (1993). "Learning medicine": The constructing of medical knowledge at Harvard Medical School. In S. Lindenbaum & M. Lock (Eds.), *Knowledge, power, and practice: The anthropology of medicine and everyday life* (pp. 81–107). University of California Press.

Grosjean, S., Farré-Coma, J., Gál, O., Laffan, A., Sendra, A., Stümpel, J., & Mestre, T. (2021). Co-designing an integrated care network with people living with Parkinson's disease: From patients' narratives to trajectory analysis. *Qualitative Health Research*, *31*(14), 2585–2601. https://doi.org/10.1177/10497323211042605

Hofmann, B. (2016). Disease, illness, and sickness. In M. Solomon, J. R. Simon, & H. Kincaid (Eds.), *The Routledge companion to philosophy of medicine* (pp. 16–26). Routledge.

Hydén, L. (1997). Illness and narrative. *Sociology of Health & Illness*, *19*(1), 48–69. https://doi.org/10.1111/j.1467-9566.1997.tb00015.x

Jackson, S. (2023). Online health communities in controversy over ME/CFS and long Covid. *European Journal of Health Communication*, *4*(2), 49–72. https://doi.org/10.47368/ejhc.2023.203

Karlsson, A., Stage, C., & Ledderer, L. (2024). Engage and withdraw: The role of peer-led online communities in the configuration of knowledge on chronic illness. *Qualitative Health Communication*, *3*(1), 4–16. https://doi.org/10.7146/qhc.138193

Khullar, D. (2022). Social media and medical misinformation: Confronting new variants of an old problem. *JAMA*, *328*(14), 1393–1394. https://doi.org/10.1001/jama.2022.17191

Killbride, M. K., & Joffe, S. (2018). The new age of patient autonomy: Implications for the patient-physician relationship. *JAMA*, *320*(19), 1973–1974. https://doi.org/10.1001/jama.2018.14382

Klawiter, M. (2004). Breast cancer in two regimes: The impact of social movements on illness experience. *Sociology of Health & Illness*, *26*(6), 845–874. https://doi.org/10.1111/j.1467-9566.2004.421_1.x

Kleinman, A. (1988). *The illness narratives: Suffering, healing, and the human condition*. Basic Books.

Krishna, A., & Thompson, T. L. (2021). Misinformation about health: A review of health communication and misinformation scholarship. *The American Behavioral Scientist*, *65*(2), 316–332. https://doi.org/10.1177/0002764219878223

Lee, S. (2023). Enregistering mask-wearing in the time of a public health crisis. *Language in Society*, *52*(3), 485–509. https://doi.org/10.1017/S0047404522000033

Lopes, F., Araújo, R., Alves, F., & Duarte, R. (2023). COVID-19 in Portugal: A pandemic redesigned by the media. *Journal of Health Communication*, *28*(sup2), 87–98. https://doi.org/10.1080/10810730.2023.2231882

López-Rico, C. M., González-Esteban, J. L., & Hernández-Martínez, A. (2020). Consumo de información en redes sociales durante la crisis de la Covid-19 en España [Information consumption in social networks during the Covid-19's crisis in Spain]. *Revista de Comunicación y Salud*, *10*(2), 461–481. https://doi.org/10.35669/rcys.2020.10(2).461–481

Lovari, A. (2020). Spreading (dis)trust: Covid-19 misinformation and government intervention in Italy. *Media and Communication*, *8*(2), 458–461. https://doi.org/10.17645/mac.v8i2.3219

Lupton, D. (2014). The commodification of patient opinion: The digital patient experience economy in the age of big data. *Sociology of Health & Illness*, *36*(6), 856–869. https://doi.org/10.1111/1467-9566.12109

Lupton, D. (2016). *The quantified self: A sociology of self-tracking*. Polity Press.

Lupton, D. (2018). *Digital health: Critical and cross-disciplinary perspectives*. Routledge.

Lupton, D. (2022). The quantified pandemic: Digitised surveillance, containment and care in response to the COVID-19 crisis. In S. Pink, M. Berg, D. Lupton, & M. Ruckenstein (Eds.), *Everyday automation: Experiencing and anticipating emerging technologies* (pp. 59–72). Routledge.

Lupton, D., & Maslen, S. (2017). Telemedicine and the senses: A review. *Sociology of Health & Illness*, *39*(8), 1557–1571. https://doi.org/10.1111/1467-9566.12617

Magnussen, H. J., Kjeken, I., Pinxsterhuis, I., Sjøvold, T. A., & Feiring, M. (2024). Dialogued into being: Constructing knowledge about hand osteoarthritis from a polyphony of voices in healthcare encounters. *International Journal of Qualitative Studies on Health and Well-being*, *19*(1), 2330221. https://doi.org/10.1080/17482631.2024.2330221

Maslen, S., & Lupton, D. (2019). "Keeping It Real": Women's enactments of lay health knowledges and expertise on Facebook. *Sociology of Health & Illness*, *41*(8), 1637–1651. https://doi.org/10.1111/1467-9566.12982

Mather, C. A., & Cummings, E. (2019). Developing and sustaining digital professionalism: A model for assessing readiness of healthcare environments and capability of nurses. *BMJ Health & Care Informatics*, *26*(1), e100062. https://doi.org/10.1136/bmjhci-2019-100062

Matusitz, J., & Breen, G. (2007). E-health: A new kind of telemedicine. *Social Work in Public Health*, *23*(1), 95–113. https://doi.org/10.1300/J523v23n01_06

May, C. (2006). The hard work of being ill. *Chronic Illness*, *2*(3), 161–162. https://doi.org/10.1177/17423953060020030701

Mazanderani, F., Locock, L., & Powell, J. (2013). Biographical value: Towards a conceptualisation of the commodification of illness narratives in contemporary healthcare. *Sociology of Health & Illness*, *35*(6), 891–905. https://doi.org/10.1111/1467-9566.12001

Memenga, P., Eitze, S., Shamsrizi, P., Addo, M. M., & Betsch, C. (2022). Debunking misinformation and communicating critical events in vaccine trials: Experimental evidence on vaccination intentions in SARS-CoV-2 pandemic. *European Journal of Health Communication*, *3*(2), 64–96. https://doi.org/10.47368/ejhc.2022.204

OECD/EU. (2022). *Health at a glance: Europe 2022. State of health in the EU cycle*. OECD Publishing.

Parviainen, J., & Rantala, J. (2022). Chatbot breakthrough in the 2020s? An ethical reflection on the trend of automated consultations in health care. *Medicine, Health Care and Philosophy*, *25*(1), 61–71. https://doi.org/10.1007/s11019-021-10049-w

Ressler, P. K., Bradshaw, Y. S., Gualtieri, L., & Chui, K. K. H. (2012). Communicating the experience of chronic pain and illness through blogging. *Journal of Medical Internet Research*, *14*(5), e143. https://doi.org/10.2196/jmir.2002

Rodgers, K., & Massac, N. (2020). Misinformation: A threat to the public's health and the public health system. *Journal of Public Health Management and Practice*, *26*(3), 294–296. https://doi.org/10.1097/PHH.0000000000001163

Rodríguez-González, A. (2021). Educación para la salud, prevención y promoción comunitaria a través de la página de Facebook de un centro de salud de atención primaria [Health education, prevention and community promotion through the Facebook page of a primary care health center]. *Revista Española de Comunicación en Salud*, *12*(1), 58–66. https://doi.org/10.20318/recs.2021.5307

Rodríguez-González, A. (2023). Conocimientos de la población sobre las medidas de prevención y detección de COVID-19: análisis de los comentarios en una publicación en la red social Facebook [Knowledge of the population about prevention and detection measures for COVID-19: Analysis of comments on a publication on the social network Facebook]. *Revista Española de Comunicación en Salud*, *14*(2), 34–45. https://doi.org/10.20318/recs.2023.7470

Rushforth, A., Ladds, E., Wieringa, S., Taylor, S., Husain, L., & Greenhalgh, T. (2021). Long Covid – the illness narratives. *Social Science & Medicine*, *286*, 114326. https://doi.org/10.1016/j.socscimed.2021.114326

Schaller, S., Wiedicke, A., Reifegerste, D., & Temmann, L. J. (2023). (De)Stigmatizing depression on social media: The role of responsibility frames. *Journal of Health Communication*, *28*(11), 757–767. https://doi.org/10.1080/10810730.2023.2266702

Sendra, A., & Farré, J. (2020). Communicating the experience of chronic pain through social media: Patients' narrative practices on Instagram. *Journal of Communication in Healthcare*, *13*(1), 46–54. https://doi.org/10.1080/17538068.2020.1752982

Sendra, A., Grosjean, S., & Bonneville, L. (2022). Co-constructing experiential knowledge in health: The contribution of people living with Parkinson to the co-design approach. *Qualitative Health Communication*, *1*(1), 101–121. https://doi.org/10.7146/qhc.v1i1.124110

Sendra, A., Torkkola, S., & Parviainen, J. (2023). Non-knowledge in medical practices: Approaching the uses of social media in healthcare from an epistemological perspective. *Journal of Digital Social Research*, *5*(1), 70–89. https://doi.org/10.33621/jdsr.v5i1.152

Sendra, A., Torkkola, S., & Parviainen, J. (2024). AstraZeneca vaccine controversies in the media: Theorizing about the mediatization of ignorance in the context of the COVID-19 vaccination campaign. *Health Communication*, *39*(3), 541–551. https://doi.org/10.1080/10410236.2023.2171951

Sola-Pueyo, J. D. (2022). La ciencia y los científicos como fuentes informativas de los medios: Análisis y aprendizajes de la pandemia del coronavirus [Science and scientists as media information sources: Analysis and learnings from the Coronavirus pandemic]. *Revista Española de Comunicación en Salud*, *13*(1), 33–45. https://doi.org/10.20318/recs.2022.6361

Sosnowy, C. (2014). Practicing patienthood online: Social media, chronic illness, and lay expertise. *Societies*, *4*(2), 316–329. https://doi.org/10.3390/soc4020316

Stage, C., Karlsson, A., & Ledderer, L. (2024). Online patient work: On the use of peer-led online communities to process and prevent discontinuity of care. *European Journal of Health Communication*, *5*(2), 44–59. https://doi.org/10.47368/ejhc.2024.203

Timmermans, S. (2020). The engaged patient: The relevance of patient-physician communication for twenty-first-century health. *Journal of Health and Social Behavior*, *61*(3), 259–273. https://doi.org/10.1177/0022146520943514

Torkkola, S. (2016a). Lääkeneuvoja sosiaalisesta mediasta [Medical advice from social media]. *SIC!*, *2016*(1), 50–52. https://urn.fi/URN:NBN:fi-fe201603098672

Torkkola, S. (2016b). Multifaceted health communication. In V. Marinescu & B. Mitu (Eds.), *Health and the media: Essays on the effects of mass communication* (pp. 17–31). McFarland & Company, Inc.

Torkkola, S., Tyni, P., Parviainen, J., & Sendra, A. (2024). Terveydenhuollon muuttuvat viestintäkäytännöt: Kyselytutkimus terveydenhuollon asiantuntijoille sosiaalisen median mahdollisuuksista ja uhista potilastyössä [Changing practices in healthcare communication: A survey for healthcare experts about opportunities and threats of social media in patient care]. *Media & Viestintä*, *47*(4), 53–78. https://doi.org/10.23983/mv.130759

Turner, B. S. (1987). *Medical power and social knowledge*. SAGE Publications.

Van Dijck, J., & Alinejad, D. (2020). Social media and trust in scientific expertise: Debating the COVID-19 pandemic in the Netherlands. *Social Media + Society*, *6*(4). https://doi.org/10.1177/2056305120981057

Varey, S., Dixon, M., Hernández, A., Mateus, C., Palmer, T. M., & Milligan, C. (2021). The role of combinatorial health technologies in supporting older people with long-term conditions: Responsibilisation or co-management of healthcare?. *Social Science & Medicine*, *269*, 113545. https://doi.org/10.1016/j.socscimed.2020.113545

Williams, G. (1984). The genesis of chronic illness: Narrative re-construction. *Sociology of Health and Illness*, *6*(2), 175–200. https://doi.org/10.1111/1467-9566.ep10778250

Wright, K. B. (2016). Communication in health-related online social support groups/communities: A review of research on predictors of participation, applications of social support theory, and health outcomes. *Review of Communication Research*, *4*, 65–87. https://www.rcommunicationr.org/index.php/rcr/article/view/42

4 From the medical gaze to the digital gaze

The history of medicine has often been described as discovering the history of diseases (see, e.g., Porter, 1999). This understanding of the history of diseases has been criticized; it has been pointed out that, although disease could be seen as a biological manifestation of ill health, it does not mean that it has remained the same throughout the centuries and across cultures (Sontag, 2002; Strong, 1998; Torkkola, 2008, pp. 17–19). One example of a socioculturally constructed disease is the difference between treatments of uterine fibroids, one of the most common gynaecological diseases (Ierardi et al., 2018). A documentary book titled *Medicine and Culture: Notions of Health and Sickness in Britain, the U.S., France and West Germany* written by journalist Lynn Payer (1996) reflects on these differences. The book is a description of the interaction between disease and culture. Diseases are interpreted through the prism of culture, which explains why a disease diagnosed identically is not treated in the same way in different countries (Payer, 1996). In the book, Payer (1996, pp. 21–22) uses as an example her own health problem, uterine fibroids, and explains the different recommendations for treatment that she received in France and the USA. In the USA, the recommended treatment was hysterectomy, whereas in France the recommendation was myectomy (Payer, 1996).

Although Payer's book was published in 1989, the core idea of the book is still valid these days, and the example of uterine fibroids still works. Recently published studies have shown that non-medical factors influence hysterectomy rates among countries with similar demographics (Edler et al., 2017), including the socio-economic status of patients (Materia, 2002) and different diagnostic practices, which are not only driven by medical factors (Veerus et al., 2015). The cultural differences not only manifest in disease treatment practices; there are also variances between the guidelines for general practitioners on the same well-defined clinical entity, which are driven by cultural factors, such as the mixture of beliefs of patients and practitioners, local habits, the influence of medical experts from hospital-based disciplines, the expectations of patients, historical evolutions in medical practice, and the organization of care (Christiaens et al., 2004).

DOI: 10.4324/9781003519607-4

Likewise, there is no common general terminology for medicine based on information technology. Researchers typically use the terms "digital medicine", "digital health", "e-health", "m-health", "medicine 2.0", and "telemedicine" in their articles (Babaei et al., 2024; Eysenbach, 2008; Fatehi & Wootton, 2012; Iyawa et al., 2016; Merrell, 2015; Zhou et al., 2024). For us, the term "infomedicine" initially sounded usable because it fits together with the word biomedicine. "Infomedicine" as a term was launched in the 1980s by Laurence Foss and Kenneth Rothenberg (1987). Unfortunately, the definition of "infomedicine" in *The Second Medical Revolution, from Biomedicine to Infomedicine* (Foss & Rothenberg, 1987) has nothing to do with telemedicine, but it refers to an infomedical model that includes not only bio-messages but also psycho- and socio-messages (Foss & Rothenberg, 1987, p. 298). Alternatively, the commonly used concept of telemedicine is defined as the use of information and communication technology in the medical practice of diagnosing, treating, and preventing diseases (Babaei et al., 2024, p. 38). However, in this book, we follow the work of Nasib Babaei et al. (2024), who use the term "virtual care". To make it wider, we have adjusted the term "virtual care" to "virtual medicine" to also include medical actions not directly connected to the care of patients, like education, training, research, and administration. The term "virtual medicine" is more suitable for the discussion on digital healthcare communication. Under this adjusted term, telemedicine and telehealth are sub-concepts of virtual medicine, which refer to concrete online medical practices.

In this chapter, we discuss the construction of disease in the digital era and the relationship between medical disease and patients. The chapter is divided as follows. First, we outline the starting point, the birth of modern medicine. Next, we describe how the digitalization of medicine reconstructs medicine as science and medicine as art – i.e., medical practice. Finally, we draw conclusions on how these changes reconstruct both care provider–care receiver interactions and patienthood and ask for a reorientation of healthcare communication.

4.1 The birth of modern medicine

Our starting point for this chapter is Michel Foucault's (1963/1994) understanding of modern medicine. As Nicholas Rose points out, the relevance of Foucault is not to history itself but to the reorientation of medical history that invites us to see

> clinical medicine as merely one component in a complex of forms of thought and practice which question aspects of individual and group life from the point of view of health, and in relation to which medical knowledges, medical experts and medical practices play a variety of different roles (1994, p. 50).

In the context of digital healthcare communication, this is an invitation to see how digitalization alters the interaction between medical and other actors, starting with doctor–patient interactions.

In *The Birth of the Clinic* (Foucault, 1963/1994), Foucault describes how the formation of biomedicine transformed patients from being sufferers of an illness to carriers of an illness. The patient, as understood today, was constructed hand in hand with modern medicine, which, in the eighteenth century, placed patients under the medical gaze and made the human body act as a surface for diseases or an object to inspect, examine, and analyse. Patients' suffering and symptoms led to a greater focus not on medicine but on the bodily anomalies that the symptoms may indicate (Foucault, 1963/1994). Hospitals collecting patients under the medical gaze enabled the development of modern medicine, also producing changes in doctor–patient relationships (Armstrong, 1983, 1994). The changes in patienthood following the birth of modern medicine are not driven by doctors, who have dominated, subjugated, and objectified the patient, but by medical technology coupled with the anonymous gaze (Armstrong, 1994, pp. 23–24). As Thomas Osborne (1994, p. 32) points out,

> Foucault associates the clinical revolution of the eighteenth century with the convergence of new forms of observation of patients (associated with hospital structures, in situ education, etc.) and the correlation of symptoms of patients in hospital with the findings of pathological anatomy.

The clinic stands as a certain kind of discursive constellation that enables the medical gaze, a new form of observation that combines the perception of disease, clinical discovery, diagnosis, and teaching at the bedside (Foucault, 1963/1994, pp. 107–124; see also Osborne, 1994, pp. 34–35). For us, Foucault's clinic and the medical gaze are starting points for understanding the reconstruction of patienthood in modern medicine. However, we are fully conscious of the critique of Foucault in which the clinical gaze as well as the doctor–patient relationship are understood as being more complex (see, e.g., Bleakley & Bligh, 2009). Furthermore, the clinic as the birthplace of modern medicine allows us to see the importance of spatiality and respatiality not only for the construction of patienthood but also for understanding communication as a part of the entity of that construction.

Although current healthcare services are more multi-professional and care providers are not only physicians (Weiner, 2012), the core of patienthood is still based on doctor–patient interactions rooted in the birth of modern medicine and the clinic. However, to understand the doctor–patient interaction, we also need to recognize the two sides of medicine: science and art (Gadamer, 1993, pp. 92–102; 1996, pp. 121–132). Hans-George Gadamer (1996, p. 95) remarks on how the science and art of medicine have become peculiarly interfused. The act of the doctor treating the patient is not typical of modern science, wherein a case is based on a rule or law (Gadamer, 1996). For the doctor, a case is, on the one hand, a particular instance of medicine and, on the other hand, a patient feeling ill (Gadamer, 1996). Thus, a consultation between the doctor and patient involves two kinds of expertise (i.e., medicine and experiential knowledge), and experiential knowledge meets both medical knowledge and medical practice. However, the distinction between science and art in medicine needs to be understood theoretically, as they are intertwined inseparably in reality. These intertwined sides of medicine are clearly seen in evidence-based medicine, which gives the best available external evidence in the care of individual patients but does not concretely dictate decisions in individual cases (Mathew, 2023).

In relation to virtual medicine, this chapter addresses how the respatialization of the medical gaze changes interactions between the care provider and care receiver. We ask how the digitalization of healthcare changes medical knowledge and medical practice. If the clinic does not frame doctor–patient interactions and the doctor does not meet the patient carrying bodily anomalies (i.e., signs of disease) but inspects those signs in digital form, what does this mean for the understanding of disease and for the entity of ill health? Furthermore, the digitalization of healthcare also frees patients from the clinic, where patients are placed under the medical gaze. What does this freedom from the clinic and the medical gaze mean for the patient and patient communication? Is it really freedom from the medical gaze, or has the gaze just altered, with the patient now simply under a virtual gaze?

4.2 Digitalization of medical information delivery

Healthcare digitalization has enabled the collection of massive amounts of electronic data about health and well-being that may give healthcare professionals, teams, and organizations a better understanding of care delivery and outcomes (Janssen et al., 2024). For care providers, the use of digital healthcare services and particularly artificial intelligence (AI) facilitates accessing, storing, and analysing information (Tokuç & Varol, 2023). Information technology expands opportunities to handle big data that cannot be dealt with manually (Gillies, 2025, pp. 405–406). For example, SNOMED CT – i.e., the systematically organized computer-processable collection of medical terms – offers a much more detailed classification scheme for diseases than the manually used disease classification ICD-10, which includes 10,760 distinct disease classifications (Gillies, 2025). SNOMED CT offers a coding scheme with over 300,000 concepts, over a million descriptions, and 1.5 million relationships (Gillies, 2025). The management of medical information through AI may reduce the professional burden on doctors and prompt the new allocation of medical work (Gillies, 2025).

According to Anita Ho (2023), AI in healthcare is used in four broad ways: monitoring users' daily activities, determining health risks, diagnosing, and determining treatment. Both AI and digital healthcare services enable care and particularly self-care outside of hospitals and clinics, promoting both patient empowerment and the responsibility of care (Ho, 2023; Merrell, 2015). However, the use of AI has been controversial in medical practice. On the one hand, using AI to control and use information could free up time for interactions between the care provider and care receiver, thus increasing the human side of medicine (Ho, 2023; Tokuç & Varol, 2023). On the other hand, the use of AI could demand more attention from care providers, thus decreasing care provider–care receiver interactions and patient empowerment (Ho, 2023). Furthermore, AI directly providing medical knowledge to the patient through a smartphone might undermine the privileged status of doctors concerning medical knowledge and reshape the traditional dynamics of knowledge and power in healthcare (Song et al., 2025).

In addition to AI, electronic medical recording has opened a new way of sharing healthcare documents between patients and healthcare professionals (Rivière et al., 2024). There are new opportunities for both physicians and patients to use electronic patient-related data. For example, electronic health records (EHRs) enable the use of question-and-answer (Q&A) systems, assisting physicians in decision-making, and enabling patients to have a better understanding of their medical history (Bardhan et al., 2024). Furthermore, the expertise of patients, which has traditionally been based on the experience of illness, is changing due to digital platforms that provide medical information to laypeople, thus creating more medically informed patients. On the one hand, these more medically informed patients might focus on discussing detailed, perhaps irrelevant biomedical research results rather than the values and preferences that are important for follow-up treatment (Hopstaken et al., 2021). On the other hand, such patients might be more capable of participating in care discussions, which in turn may increase the quality of care (Hopstaken et al., 2021).

Medical information, increasingly distributed through the Internet and utilized by patients, causes conflicts in doctor–patient relationships. This is because doctors not only manage patients with more access to medical information, but also patients have increased embodied knowledge (Sendra et al., 2023) of situations that might lead to different constructions of disease. For doctors, the informed patient is sometimes perceived as a source of uncomfortable knowledge (Rayner, 2012), especially when the informed patient is highlighting their non-knowledge (Raz, 2024; Sendra et al., 2023). In this context, Barker et al. (2024, p. 204) explain that "to create a diagnostic category is to wrestle with and, to some extent, tame ignorance". Table 4.1, which was developed by both authors and Jaana Parviainen in a previous study, shows from a theoretical perspective some of the strategies that doctors might engage in if they perceive that non-knowledge is compromising their authority, in this case regarding embodied knowledge generated through social media. However, evidence indicates that the management of medical ignorance seems to be a

Table 4.1 Doctors' management of embodied knowledge generated through social media. Definitions paraphrased from Rayner (2012); examples provided by Sendra et al. (2023). Adapted from "Non-Knowledge in Medical Practices: Approaching the Uses of Social Media in Healthcare From an Epistemological Perspective", by A. Sendra, S. Torkkola, and J. Parviainen, 2023, *Journal of Digital Social Research*, 5(1), 75. https://doi.org/10.33621/jdsr.v5i1.152. CC BY-SA.

Strategy	*Definition*	*Application example*
Denial	Uncomfortable knowledge is totally refused	Doctors do not acknowledge patients' knowledge generated through social media
Dismissal	It is admitted that uncomfortable knowledge exists, but then it is also refused for reasons such as unreliability or lack of precision	Doctors acknowledge patients' knowledge generated through social media, but the information is later discarded by citing misinformation concerns
Diversion	A distraction is created to get away from the uncomfortable knowledge	Doctors invite patients to consult other informational resources, such as scientific papers
Displacement	A distraction is created to avoid uncomfortable knowledge and alternatives are placed	Informational resources recommended by doctors become alternatives to knowledge generated through social media

practice embedded in the diagnostic process of the disease (Barker et al., 2024; Raz, 2024). As Raz (2024, Discussion section, para. 5) points out, "biomedical science not only produces knowledge but ignores or excludes knowledge that contradicts its paradigm". The digitalization of healthcare communication has made these dynamics around non-knowledge take on greater importance, calling for the development of new medical practices that better consider the unknowns of medicine.

The digital delivery of information has also increased access to medical dis- and misinformation, generating concerns among medical authorities and healthcare professionals since the dawn of the Internet (Afful-Dadzie et al., 2023; Malik et al., 2023). Misinformation topics concerning health are wide, even though some are more common than others. According to a systematic review by Suarez-Liedo and Alvarez-Galvez (2021), issues related to smoking and drugs have the highest rate of misinformation. Misinformation related to vaccines, diet or eating disorders, noncommunicable diseases, and pandemics and communicable diseases is also common (Suarez-Liedo & Alvarez-Galvez, 2021). The lowest levels of health misinformation are related to medical treatments (Suarez-Liedo & Alvarez-Galvez, 2021). The power of social media in relation to medical dis- and misinformation reached a peak during the COVID-19 pandemic. The Director-General of the WHO (2021) summed it up in a statement in which the WHO warned that "we are not just fighting an epidemic, but an infodemic". Studies on social media and COVID-19 have shown that the motivation for sharing dis- and misinformation arises from anxiety, fear, or COVID-19 perceived risks, but entertainment, information-seeking, socialization, self-promotion, lack of trust in science, lack of self-efficacy, and altruism are also reasons for spreading dis- and misinformation (Malik et al., 2023).

During the pandemic, rumours, stigma, and conspiracy theories operated against evidence-based guidelines, a situation that might have had serious implications for public health (Islam et al., 2020). To decrease the effects of dis- and misinformation, it is seen as important that governments and international health agencies continue to deliver correct information (Islam et al., 2020). Furthermore, healthcare professionals, especially physicians, have been asked to be active on social media and follow what kind of information is used on these online platforms, direct laypeople to reliable sources of information, educate people in evaluating the quality of medical information sources, and actively diminish the spread of low-quality information (Afful-Dadzie et al., 2023). However, for healthcare professionals, an active presence on social media can cause negative experiences, even hostile actions (Grimes et al., 2020). Consequently, many healthcare professionals may avoid an open presence on these online platforms (Torkkola et al., 2024). As explained in previous chapters (see Chapter 2), the difficulties with mis- and disinformation sometimes materialize also in the medical consultation.

This process of digitalization is changing medical education and simultaneously requiring the further training of healthcare professionals. Video games, augmented reality, and other online platforms (Baashar et al., 2022; Hamilton, 2005; Losh, 2007) move medical education from the bedside of the patient at the clinic (Beigzadeh et al., 2019) to online learning environments without real patients. The learning outcomes of this new form of education are mixed. On the positive side, online learning can improve performance time, confidence, and satisfaction, but there is no clear evidence in relation to online learning and the improvement of knowledge and skills (Baashar et al., 2022; Hamilton, 2005; Kononowicz et al., 2019). In earlier studies, there was also negative feedback because of the inability to interact with other students, which resulted in perceiving computer-based learning as a poor substitute for teaching clinical skills with lecturers (Hamilton, 2005).

Likewise, these virtual environments not only offer new conditions for learning but also reconstruct professionalism, patienthood, and the relationship between the care provider and care receiver. For example, in the video game *Immune Attack*, a patient is invited to become a paraprofessional serving as the subject of their own experiment (Losh, 2007), changing the patient's traditional experience based on illness to an experience more based on medical knowledge. Additionally, there are also non-profit games designed for crisis-training professionals (Losh, 2007). In these games, crisis managers and their associated official institutions are presented in a positive and collegial light, while victims of the crisis and potential patients are presented as irritable, panicked, or uncooperative (Losh, 2007).

4.3 Digitalization of medical care

In spite of public discussion on the empowerment of the patient (Affinito et al., 2022; Calvillo et al., 2015), the idea of the patient lying on the bed remains culturally dominant. This dominance is not so often spoken out loud, but it is commonly represented in the visualization of patienthood, demonstrated by the images below (see Torkkola, 2008, pp. 235–239). In a typical photo of health-related news, the patient is placed lying on the bed, often also under the gaze of the surrounding doctors (see Figure 4.1). This visualization of patienthood might be driven by *The Anatomy Lesson of Dr. Nicolaes Tulp*,

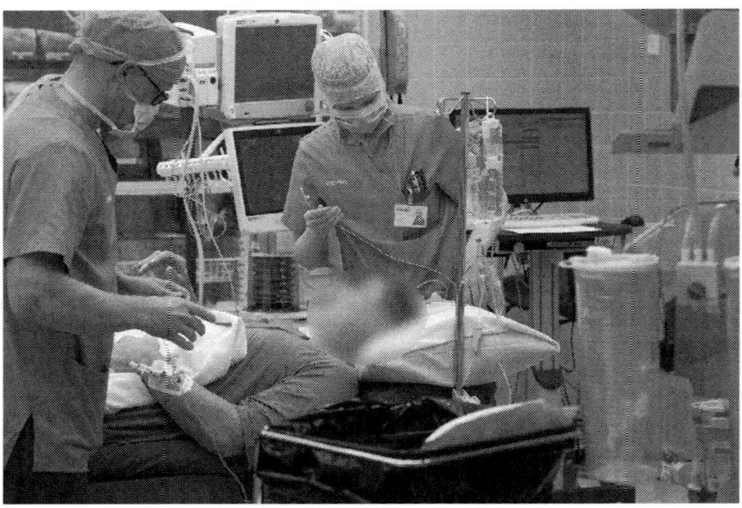

Figure 4.1 Example of the visualization of patienthood featured in the Finnish newspaper *Aamulehti*. The image has been converted to greyscale, and the patient's face has been blurred for the purposes of this publication. From "Matin uusi lonkka [Matti's new hip]", by V. Vanhalakka (text) and O. Ahola (photo and video), April 23, 2023, *Aamulehti* (https://www.aamulehti.fi/tampere/art–2000009445720.html). Photograph by Ossi Ahola for *Aamulehti* (© 2023). Reprinted with permission.

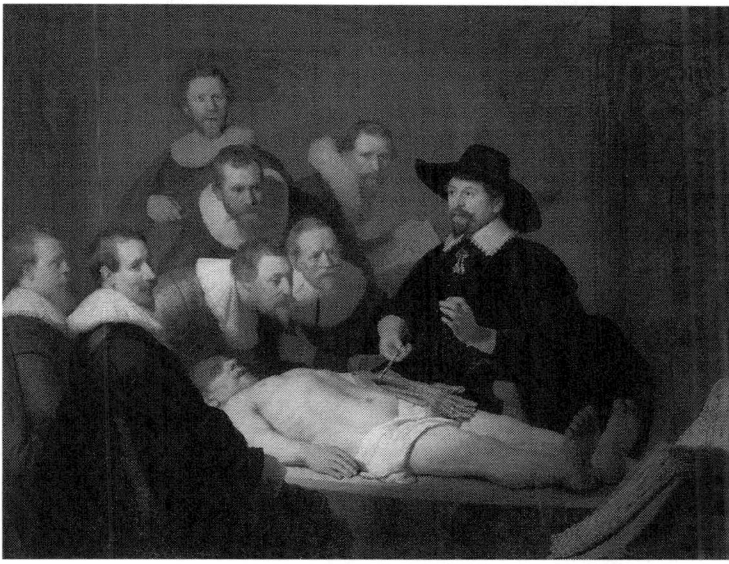

Figure 4.2 *The Anatomy Lesson of Dr. Nicolaes Tulp*. The image has been converted to greyscale for the purposes of this publication. From *The Anatomy Lesson of Dr. Nicolaes Tulp* [Oil painting] by Rembrandt, 1632, Wikipedia (https://commons.wikimedia.org/wiki/File:Rembrandt_-_The_Anatomy_Lesson_of_Dr_Nicolaes_Tulp.jpg#/media/File:Rembrandt_-_The_Anatomy_Lesson_of_Dr_Nicolaes_Tulp.jpg). Public domain.

painted by Rembrandt in 1632 (see Figure 4.2). Other examples of this type of health-related news photos include the cover of *Der Spiegel* from the issue 51/2016 titled "In der Krankenfabrik" ("In the Sick Factory") (Der Spiegel, 2016) or the photo accompanying a news piece on cancer treatment in Afghanistan featured in the Spanish newspaper *El País* (Vilà, 2022). In the coming years, when physicians and other healthcare professionals interact more virtually with patients and face-to-face contacts are less common (Weiner, 2012), the visual order of patienthood might be reconstructed, too.

The simple mantra of whatever, wherever, and whenever, typically associated with telemedicine (Merrell, 2015), distils the reorientation of digital healthcare services and virtual medical practices. However, telemedicine is not as novel as we might think. As a practice, telemedicine was probably used for the first time when a Dutch physician utilized the telephone for transmitting and monitoring heart sounds in 1905 (Bashshur et al., 2013; Fathi et al., 2017). In 1936, the telephone and the television were named as future tools for doctors in an article published in the *British Medical Journal* (Brown & Webster, 2004,

p. 86). In spite of those historical roots, modern telemedicine was established in the 1990s (Tariq et al., 2021), with its use increasing significantly all over the world during the COVID-19 pandemic (Tariq et al., 2021). Virtual medicine is not only about reordering the clinic but also about reordering the bodies and the diseases carried on the bodies (Brown & Webster, 2004, pp. 81–104). In her ethnography study, Annette Mol (2002) describes how one disease, atherosclerosis, spreads out in the hospital, thus becoming an object that enacts multiple practices instead of being an object located in one place and carried by one patient. Therefore, when a disease is not a single object found in the body, the gaze trying to see an object on the patient's body transforms into a gaze trying to follow the objects that are constructed in the multiple medical practices of healthcare professionals (Mol, 2002, p. 159). Thus, when trying to understand the digitalization of disease, we need to understand how disease is communicated through the complex practices where a disease is enacted and how these practices respatialize and retemporalize disease and its care. The culmination point of virtual medicine is that a patient searching for or receiving care does not meet a care provider in person in the clinic. This is the most remarkable change in relation to communication in healthcare, where interaction between the care provider and care receiver has been based on in-person interaction onsite for hundreds of years.

Virtual healthcare services carry a wide variety of clinical applications for remote diagnosis and treatment, as well as the supporting functions of these applications, like documentation and the exchange of health and medical information, physician order entry protocols, and patient and provider education and research (Bashshur et al., 2013). The functions of virtual healthcare services include storage and forwarding of information, interactive services, remote care receiver monitoring, teleconsultation, and guided self-help (WHO, 2023). Virtual healthcare can be divided into three categories: synchronous telehealth, asynchronous telehealth, and remote monitoring.

In synchronous telehealth, the care provider and care receiver have a live discussion online via telephone, videophone, videoconference, or consultation application (Byambasuren et al., 2023; WHO, 2023). In its simplest form, synchronous telehealth is a consultation through a phone between a care provider and a care receiver, which has been used for decades (Bashshur et al., 2013). Currently, besides phone calls and video calls, there are plenty of online platforms and applications where the care provider and care receiver can interact in real time (see, e.g., De Moraes et al., 2022; Gao et al., 2025; Lin et al., 2022).

Asynchronous telehealth is the transmission of medical data, like images, notes, and videos, to the care provider (Moreno-Ramírez & Argenziano, 2017; WHO, 2023). However, it also includes written interactions between the care provider and care receiver through e-mail (Newhouse et al., 2015; Nordtug et al., 2021), written communication through applications or platforms (Bardhan et al., 2024; Gao et al., 2025), and even technical communication through said applications, like the renewal of electronic prescriptions (Oravainen et al.,

2021; Zadeh & Tremblay, 2016). The retemporalization of care is manifested in asynchronous telehealth, where, instead of simultaneous consultation hours, care providers and care receivers calibrate their own time (Grønning et al., 2024). E-mail consultations, for instance, open a permanent (latent) written contact between the doctor and patient that changes the division of care and invites the patient to be a co-producer of social relations and healthcare (Grønning et al., 2024).

Likewise, remote monitoring offers a way for the care provider to observe patients' physiological parameters remotely and to intervene if abnormalities appear (Serrano et al., 2023). Remote monitoring applications are particularly used for chronic disease follow-ups, such as chronic kidney disease (Ghozali et al., 2023), diabetes (Andrès et al., 2019), hypertension (Zhou et al., 2024), and cardiac patients with pacemakers (Raes et al., 2024), but also for antenatal care and pregnancy monitoring (Mohamed et al., 2025). Furthermore, telemonitoring invites patients to share the responsibility for care (Ekstedt et al., 2023). The mutual engagement of patients and healthcare professionals in telemonitoring and managing disease symptoms together is an elementary part of patient safety (Ekstedt et al., 2023). In a review of studies on the transformation of patient–physician communication between 1999 and 2023 by Song et al. (2025), three main topics were found: (1) the patient–physician relationship and shared decision-making, (2) patient empowerment and education strategies, and (3) healthcare systems and health IT implementations. The first and second topics (i.e., decision-making and empowerment) are strongly rooted in communication actions and a mutual understanding of what is subject to decision-making and why those options are available for choosing. Mutual understanding may become more complicated because of the extension of the sources of medical information. In other words, a clinician making a clinical decision based on evidence-based medicine could face a patient with other kinds of information (see Mitchell, 2011).

Compared to other elements of virtual medicine, onsite doctor–patient interactions are seen as the most demanding to transform into online communication. In modern medicine, the diagnosis is not solely based on vision; touch, hearing, and smell have all been important aspects of medical care, which are difficult to replace by technical sensors (Lupton & Maslen, 2017). Rooted in embodied doctors, the art of care and the humanistic side of medicine have been central to the profession for more than two thousand years (Tokuç & Varol, 2023). Patients have traditionally relied on having the doctor by their bedside, and that is more difficult to replace with technology than accessing, storing, and analysing medical information (Tokuç & Varol, 2023). Most of the emotional communication occurs non-verbally through tone of voice, body posture, gaze, and eye contact, and this is difficult to enact through online communication (Ritunga et al., 2024). However, these communication components that are missing in online consultation can be implemented through the verbalization of empathy (Ritunga et al., 2024). For example, in written communication, oralizations are a way to express communication acts that are hard to code in neutral typed text (Nordtug et al., 2021).

Similarly, virtual medicine can be organized not only in the interaction between a care provider and care receiver; it can also happen without the intervention of any care provider. For instance, self-help digital mental health interventions (self-help DMHIs) are one example of treatment without the intervention of healthcare professionals (Fitzpatrick et al., 2024). In mental healthcare self-help, DMHIs have been developed to respond to an access crisis to psychotherapeutic interventions, although the promising expectations have been met only partly because too little attention has been paid to the views of users (Fitzpatrick et al., 2024).

Usability, privacy concerns, and digital literacy are some of the main barriers hindering the use of digital technologies for promoting shared decision-making and patient empowerment (Song et al., 2025). Access to health records is a key element for participating in decision-making. However, the right to read one's own health record has not always been self-evident, with physicians predicting negative consequences, such as patients being frightened and confused by reading their records (Delbanco et al., 2012). In this context, there have been patient movements not only demanding access to records but also claiming the right to co-write the records (Delbanco et al., 2001). Likewise, access rights to health records vary from country to country. Although in many countries residents have access to their medical data, details vary in relation to how the data are accessed, what data are available (and from when they are available), and whether full electronic access is supported by hard law (which explicitly mandates a care provider to share the records) or by soft law (where the decision regarding which data sets may be displayed to patients is left to the discretion of regional counties, care providers, or sometimes even individual physicians) (Essén et al., 2018).

Today, the care provider and care receiver widely share the view that the digitalization of patient records has improved patients' access to records and strengthened patients' empowerment and participation in decision-making (Hopstaken et al., 2021; Thielmann et al., 2023). Besides the traditional written medical documentation, patients may have access to visual information like X-rays and ultrasounds from the body's interior that affect both the experience of illness and the patient's medical knowledge (Stacey, 1997, pp. 150–176; see also Cartwright, 1995). Access to medical records facilitates informed healthcare decision-making, prevents decisional conflict, improves communication between care providers and care receivers, and increases patient satisfaction (Hopstaken et al., 2021; Thielmann et al., 2023). However, people's readiness to accept, sign in, and use online medical records depends on their personal experience and feelings as well as on multifarious technical and sociocultural factors (Lupton, 2019). In particular, socio-demographic background factors, such as the level of digital and health literacy, affect patients' opportunities to utilize their health records and strengthen their empowerment (Song et al.,

2025; Thielmann et al., 2023). Therefore, technical access to health records is only the first step that needs to be complemented with many other factors, like digital literacy and real opportunities to use digital technologies and applications (see, e.g., Gauthier-Beaupré & Grosjean, 2023), to fulfil the necessary conditions for the implementation of the self-determination rights of citizens related to ill health.

4.4 Towards joint expertise

Virtual medicine improves both access to medical information and healthcare services (Table 4.2), which have been seen as the main advantages of virtual medicine (see, e.g., Bashshur et al., 2013; Kirby et al., 2025; Mathews et al., 2023; Ritunga et al., 2024). From the viewpoint of patients, improved access to medical information and healthcare services supports patient independence, promotes empowerment, constructs a more informed patient, and changes the care provider–care receiver relationship. Consequently, the expertise constructed in the interaction between the care provider and care receiver is altering due to the more informed patient. In this new environment, more empowered patients are no longer passive recipients of care who resign to listening to authoritative monologues; they are able to resist the power and expert authority of healthcare professionals and demand a more participatory role in their care (see, e.g., Ha & Longnecker, 2010).

Care receivers are not only users of medical information; they are also actively involved in information production. In remote monitoring, the responsibility for care is shared between the care provider and care receiver (Bolt et al., 2023; Ekstedt et al., 2023; Grønning et al., 2024). However, telemonitoring is not a tool that necessarily increases equal accessibility, good quality of

Table 4.2 Changes in the delivery of medical information and care services

Changes	*References*
Online medical information delivery and care services . . .	
. . .increases access to medical information, including mis- and disinformation	Afful-Dadzie et al. (2023), Malik et al. (2023), Suarez-Lledo and Alvarez-Galvez (2021)
. . .increases care receivers' access to their own medical records	Delbanco et al. (2001), Hopstaken et al. (2021), Thielmann et al. (2023)
. . .facilitates the move towards the shared responsibility of care	Bolt et al. (2023), Ekstedt et al. (2023), Grønning et al. (2024)
. . .permits the advance of more medically informed patients	Ho (2023), Hopstaken et al. (2021), Merrell (2015), Song et al. (2025)
. . .changes the interaction between care providers and care receivers	Ritunga et al. (2024), Song et al. (2025), Tokuç and Varol (2023)

care, and patient autonomy; the outcomes of telemonitoring are dependent on choices regarding the design of specific monitoring systems, their development process, and their embeddedness in a trusting physician–patient relationship (Bolt et al., 2023). This highlights the importance of engaging in alternative creation processes for remote monitoring systems (as well as other technologies) that better consider the patients' needs (Gauthier-Beaupré & Grosjean, 2023). The transformation of care from the clinic to the home medicalizes private spaces; that is, for the patient, virtual medicine is not only a technical change but also a change in everyday life (Leonardsen et al., 2020). Moreover, patients are invited to be more informed and active in preventing disease and promoting health (Prodović-Milojković et al., 2024). We will address the changes regarding personal responsibility for health promotion and the construction of digital health citizenship in the next chapter (Chapter 5).

Currently, the increasing demand for medical treatment is moving care from hospital wards to patients' homes, as in the case of acute care (Wilkes et al., 2024). Within decades, amid the intensification of virtual medicine, smart hospitals using AI and other digital technologies will tailor care to each patient, with specialized care also moving into the patient's home (Jovy-Klein et al., 2024). Thus, the respatialization of care will be manifested in the decreasing need for hospital buildings. It is feasible that existing enormous hospital complexes worldwide will pass into history. It is conceivable that the care of the future will be enacted in shopping centres or similar places. The individual entering the shopping centre will be scanned and then get a personalized health report and recommendations for care to be done at home, where 3D printers will produce the medications and equipment needed for individualized care. This kind of physical change will alter not only the care provider–care receiver relationship but also the entity of ill health in society.

In this chapter, we have gone through the transformation of disease from modern medicine to virtual medicine. The digitalization of healthcare has transformed modern medicine, located in the clinic and manifested by the medical gaze observing abnormalities of the body expressed in signs (i.e., symptoms of disease), into the digital gaze following signs of disease that spread out in the digital realm. Therefore, the patient lying on the bed is not an essential element of medical practice. A disease can be diagnosed without a simultaneous doctor–patient interaction, solely based on virtual signs of disease. This transformation can be seen as the end of the patient that was born hand in hand with modern medicine. However, as we saw in the previous chapter, within the digitalization of healthcare, the patient and the experience of illness have also been reconstructed, and new disease regimes where the experience of being ill from the perspective of the patient has adopted a more significant role has entered healthcare and asked for changes in care provider–care receiver interactions as well as in healthcare communication in general. In Chapter 5, we will discuss how the digitalization of healthcare transforms the relations of ill health in society.

References

Affinito, L., Fontanella, A., Montano, N., & Brucato, A. (2022). How physicians can empower patients with digital tools: A joint study of the Italian Scientific Society of Internal Medicine (FADOI) and the European Federation of Internal Medicine (EFIM). *Journal of Public Health*, *30*(4), 897–909. https://doi.org/10.1007/s10389-020-01370-4

Afful-Dadzie, E., Afful-Dadzie, A., & Egala, S. B. (2023). Social media in health communication: A literature review of information quality. *Health Information Management Journal*, *52*(1), 3–17. https://doi.org/10.1177/1833358321992683

Andrès, E., Meyer, L., Zulfiqar, A.-A., Hajjam, M., Talha, S., Bahougne, T., Ervé, S., Hajjam, J., Doucet, J., Jeandidier, N., & El Hassani, A. H. (2019). Telemonitoring in diabetes: Evolution of concepts and technologies, with a focus on results of the more recent studies. *Journal of Medicine and Life*, *12*(3), 203–214. https://pmc.ncbi.nlm.nih.gov/articles/PMC6814890/

Armstrong, D. (1983). *Political anatomy of the body: Medical knowledge in Britain in the Twentieth century*. Cambridge University Press.

Armstrong, D. (1994). Bodies of knowledge/knowledge of bodies. In C. Jones & R. Porter (Eds.), *Reassessing foucault: Power, medicine and the body* (pp. 17–27). Routledge.

Baashar, Y., Alkawsi, G., Ahmad, W. N. W., Alhussian, N., Alwadain, A., Capretz, L. F., Babiker, A., & Alghail, A. (2022). Effectiveness of using augmented reality for training in the medical professions: Meta-analysis. *JMIR Serious Games*, *10*(3), e32715. https://doi.org/10.2196/32715

Babaei, N., Zamanzadeh, V., Valizadeh, L., Lotfi, M., Kousha, A., Samad-Soltani, T., & Avazeh, M. (2024). Virtual care in the health care system: A concept analysis. *Scandinavian Journal of Caring Sciences*, *38*(1), 35–46. https://doi.org/10.1111/scs.13227

Bardhan, J., Roberts, K., & Wang, D. Z. (2024). Question answering for electronic health records: Scoping review of datasets and models. *Journal of Medical Internet Research*, *26*, e53636. https://doi.org/10.2196/53636

Barker, K. K., Whooley, O., Madden, E. F., Ahrend, E. E., & Greene, R. N. (2024). The long tail of COVID and the tale of long COVID: Diagnostic construction and the management of ignorance. *Sociology of Health & Illness*, *46*(S1), 189–207. https://doi.org/10.1111/1467-9566.13599

Bashshur, R. L., Shannon, G., Krupinski, E. A., & Grigsby, J. (2013). Sustaining and realizing the promise of telemedicine. *Telemedicine and e-Health*, *19*(5), 339–345. https://doi.org/10.1089/tmj.2012.0282

Beigzadeh, A., Adibi, P., Bahaadinbeigy, K., & Yamani, N. (2019). Strategies for teaching in clinical rounds: A systematic review of the literature. *Journal of Research in Medical Sciences*, *24*(1), 33. https://doi.org/10.4103/jrms.JRMS_460_18

Bleakley, A., & Bligh, J. (2009). Who can resist foucault? *The Journal of Medicine and Philosophy*, *34*(4), 368–383. https://doi.org/10.1093/jmp/jhp028

Bolt, I., Specker, J., & Schermer, M. (2023). Telemonitoring: Ethical lessons from the COVID-19 pandemic. *BMC Digital Health*, *1*, 47. https://doi.org/10.1186/s44247-023-00046-9

Brown, N., & Webster, A. (2004). *New medical technologies and society: Reordering life*. Polity Press.

Byambasuren, O., Greenwood, H., Bakhit, M., Atkins, T., Clark, J., Scott, A. M., & Glasziou, P. (2023). Comparison of telephone and video Telehealth consultations: Systematic review. *Journal of Medical Internet Research*, *25*, e49942. https://doi.org/10.2196/49942

Calvillo, J., Román, I., & Roa, L. M. (2015). How technology is empowering patients? A literature review. *Health Expectations*, *18*(5), 643–652. https://doi.org/10.1111/hex.12089

Cartwright, L. (1995). *Screening the body: Tracing medicine's visual culture*. University of Minnesota Press.

Christiaens, T., De Backer, D., Burgers, J., & Baerheim, A. (2004). Guidelines, evidence, and cultural factors: Comparison of four European guidelines on uncomplicated cystitis. *Scandinavian Journal of Primary Health Care*, *22*(3), 141–145. https://doi.org/10.1080/02813430410006521

De Moraes, V. Y., Ferreira, C. B., Kawagoe, C. K., Gushken, F., Azevedo, G., & Filho, M. F. (2022). An integrative telehealth platform managed by nurses. *BMC Research Notes*, *15*, 301. https://doi.org/10.1186/s13104-022-06197-8

Delbanco, T., Berwick, D. M., Boufford, J. I., Edgman-Levitan, Ollenschläger, G., Plamping, D., & Rockefeller, R. G. (2001). Healthcare in a land called PeoplePower: Nothing about me without me. *Health Expectations*, *4*(3), 144–150. https://doi.org/10.1046/j.1369-6513.2001.00145.x

Delbanco, T., Walker, J., Bell, S. K., Darer, J. D., Elmore, J. G., Farag, N., Feldman, H. J., Mejilla, R., Ngo, L., Ralston, J. D., Ross, S. E., Trivedi, N., Vodicka, E., & Leveille, S. G. (2012). Inviting patients to read their Doctors' notes: A quasi-experimental study and a look ahead. *Annals of Internal Medicine*, *157*(7), 461–470. https://doi.org/10.7326/0003-4819-157-7-201210020-00002

Der Spiegel. (2016, December 16). *In der Krankenfabrik* [In the Sick Factory]. https://www.spiegel.de/spiegel/print/index-2016–51.html

Edler, K., Tamussino, K., Fülöp, G., Reinstadler, E., Neunteufel, W., Reif, P., Laky, R., & Aigmüller, T. (2017). Rates and routes of hysterectomy for benign indications in Austria 2002–2014. *Geburtshilfe Und Frauenheilkunde*, *77*(05), 482–486. https://doi.org/10.1055/s-0043-107784

Ekstedt, M., Nordheim, E. S., Hellström, A., Strandberg, S., & Hagerman, H. (2023). Patient safety and sense of security when telemonitoring chronic conditions at home: The views of patients and healthcare professionals – a qualitative study. *BMC Health Services Research*, *23*, 581. https://doi.org/10.1186/s12913-023-09428-1

Essén, A., Scandurra, I., Gerrits, R., Humphrey, G., Johansen, M. A., Kierkegaard, P., Koskinen, J., Liaw, S.-T., Odeh, S., Ross, P., & Ancker, J. S. (2018). Patient access to electronic health records: Differences across ten countries. *Health Policy and Technology*, *7*(1), 44–56. https://doi.org/10.1016/j.hlpt.2017.11.003

Eysenbach, G. (2008). Medicine 2.0: Social networking, collaboration, participation, apomediation, and openness. *Journal of Medical Internet Research*, *10*(3), e22. https://doi.org/10.2196/jmir.1030

Fatehi, F., & Wootton, R. (2012). Telemedicine, telehealth or e-health? A bibliometric analysis of the trends in the use of these terms. *Journal of Telemedicine and Telecare*, *18*(8), 460–464. https://doi.org/10.1258/jtt.2012.gth108

Fathi, J. T., Modin, H. E., & Scott, J. D. (2017). Nurses advancing telehealth services in the era of healthcare reform. *The Online Journal of Issues in Nursing*, *22*(2), 2. https://doi.org/10.3912/OJIN.Vol22No02Man02

Fitzpatrick, S., Crenshaw, A. O., Donkin, V., Collins, A., Xiang, A., Earle, E. A., Goenka, K., Varma, S., Bushe, J., McFadden, T., Librado, A., & Monson, C. (2024). We have spent time, money, and effort making self-help digital mental health interventions: Is anyone going to come to the party?. *Journal of Medical Internet Research*, *26*, e58198. https://doi.org/10.2196/58198

Foss, L., & Rothenberg, K. (1987). *The second medical revolution. From biomedicine to infomedicine*. New Science Library.

Foucault, M. (1994). *The birth of the clinic: An archaeology of medical perception*. Vintage Books. (Original work publihsed 1963)

Gadamer, H.-G. (1993). *Uber die Verborgenheit der Gesundheit: Aufsätze und Vorträge* [On the enigma of health: Essays and lectures]. Suhrkamp.

Gadamer, H.-G. (1996). *The enigma of health: The art of healing in a scientific age*. Polity Press.

Gao, R., Feng, S.-Y., Zheng, J., Zhai, L.-J., & Liu, R. (2025). Telehealth and telemedicine in the management of adult patients after liver transplantation: A scoping review. *Telemedicine & e-Health*, *31*(4), 375–385. https://doi.org/10.1089/tmj.2024.0359

Gauthier-Beaupré, A., & Grosjean, S. (2023). Understanding acceptability of digital health technologies among francophone-speaking communities across the world: A meta-ethnographic study. *Frontiers in Communication*, *8*, 1230015. https://doi.org/10.3389/fcomm.2023.1230015

Ghozali, M. T., Satibi, S., & Forthwengel, G. (2023). The impact of mobile health applications on the outcomes of patients with chronic kidney disease: A systematic review and meta-analysis. *Journal of Medicine and Life*, *16*(9), 1299–1309. https://pmc.ncbi.nlm.nih.gov/articles/PMC10719786/

Gillies, A. (2025). *Healthcare management: Global perspectives*. Routledge.

Grimes, D. R., Brennan, L. J., & O'Connor, R. (2020). Establishing a taxonomy of potential hazards associated with communicating medical science in the age of disinformation. *BMJ Open*, *10*(7), e035626. https://doi.org/10.1136/bmjopen-2019-035626

Grønning, A., Simonsen, L. M., Lüchau, E. C., Hvidt, E. A., & Klausen, M. (2024). My time, your time, our time. Older patients' and GPs' time sensibilities around email consultations. *Health Sociology Review*, *33*(1), 43–58. https://doi.org/10.1080/14461242.2024.2316742

Ha, J. F., & Longnecker, N. (2010). Doctor–patient communication: A review. *The Ochsner Journal*, *10*(1), 38–43. https://pmc.ncbi.nlm.nih.gov/articles/PMC3096184/

Hamilton, R. (2005). Nurses' knowledge and skill retention following cardiopulmonary resuscitation training: A review of the literature. *Journal of Advanced Nursing*, *51*(3), 288–297. https://doi.org/10.1111/j.1365-2648.2005.03491.x

Ho, A. (2023). Artificial intelligence as a feminist bioethics issue. In W. A. Rogers, J. L. Scully, S. M. Carter, V. A. Entwistle, & C. Mills (Eds.), *The Routledge handbook of feminist bioethics* (pp. 291–307). Routledge.

Hopstaken, J. S., Verweij, L., Van Laarhoven, C. J. H. M., Blijlevens, N. M. A., Stommel, M. W. J., 6 Hermens, R. P. M. G. (2021). Effect of digital care platforms on quality of care for oncological patients and barriers and facilitators for their implementation: Systematic review. *Journal of Medical Internet Research*, *23*(9), e28869. https://doi.org/10.2196/28869

Ierardi, A. M., Savasi, V., Angileri, S. A., Petrillo, M., Sbaraini, S., Pinto, A., Hanozet, F., Marconi, A. M., & Carrafiello, G. (2018). Percutaneous high frequency microwave ablation of uterine fibroids: Systematic review. *BioMed Research International*, *2018*(1), 1–9. https://doi.org/10.1155/2018/2360107

Islam, M. S., Sarkar, T., Khan, S. H., Kamal, A.-H. M., Hasan, S. M. M., Kabir, A., Yeasmin, D., Islam, M. A., Chowdhury, K. I. A., Anwar, K. S., Chughtai, A. A., & Seale, H. (2020). COVID-19–related infodemic and its impact on public health: A global social media analysis. *The American Journal of Tropical Medicine and Hygiene*, *103*(4), 1621–1629. https://doi.org/10.4269/ajtmh.20-0812

Iyawa, G. E., Herselman, M., & Botha, A. (2016). Digital health innovation ecosystems: From systematic literature review to conceptual framework. *Procedia Computer Science*, *100*, 244–252. https://doi.org/10.1016/j.procs.2016.09.149

Janssen, A., Donnelly, C., & Shaw, T. (2024). A taxonomy for health information systems. *Journal of Medical Internet Research*, *26*, e47682. https://doi.org/10.2196/47682

Jovy-Klein, F., Stead, S., Salge, T. O., Sander, J., Diehl, A., & Antons, D. (2024). Forecasting the future of smart hospitals: Findings from a real-time delphi study. *BMC Health Services Research*, *24*, 1421. https://doi.org/10.1186/s12913-024-11895-z

Kirby, A., Griffin, D., Heavin, C., Drummond, F. J., McGrath, C., & Kiely, F. (2025). Telehealth adoption in palliative care: A systematic review of patient barriers and facilitators. *BMC Palliative Care*, *24*, 52. https://doi.org/10.1186/s12904-025-01698-2

Kononowicz, A. A., Woodham, L. A., Edelbring, S., Stathakarou, N., Davies, D., Saxena, N., Car, L. T., Carlstedt-Duke, J., Car, J., & Zary, N. (2019). Virtual patient simulations in health professions education: Systematic review and meta-analysis by the digital health education collaboration. *Journal of Medical Internet Research*, *21*(7), e14676. https://doi.org/10.2196/14676

Leonardsen, A.-C. L., Hardeland, C., Helgesen, A. K., & Grøndahl, V. A. (2020). Patient experiences with technology enabled care across healthcare settings - a systematic review. *BMC Health Services Research*, *20*, 779. https://doi.org/10.1186/s12913-020-05633-4

Lin, B. S., Li, Y. Y., Qiao, C., Liu, J., Wang, J., Wan, M., Lin, M. J., Zhang, W. L., Ding, Y. M., Kong, Q. Z., Duan, M., Zuo, X. L., & Li, Y. Q. (2022). Implementation of WeChat-based patient–doctor interaction in the management of *Helicobacter pylori* infection: A propensity score matching analysis. *Journal of Digestive Diseases*, *23*(5–6), 280–287. https://doi.org/10.1111/1751-2980.13114

Losh, E. (2007). Walls, doors, condoms, and duct tape: Serious games about national security and public health. *Discourse*, *29*(1), 101–119. https://doi.org/10.1353/dis.2007.a252908

Lupton, D. (2019). 'I'd like to think you could trust the government, but I don't really think we can': Australian women's attitudes to and experiences of My Health Record. *Digital Health*, *5*. https://doi.org/10.1177/2055207619847017

Lupton, D., & Maslen, S. (2017). Telemedicine and the senses: A review. *Sociology of Health & Illness*, *39*(8), 1557–1571. https://doi.org/10.1111/1467-9566.12617

Malik, A., Bashir, F., & Mahmood, K. (2023). Antecedents and consequences of misinformation sharing behavior among adults on social media during COVID−19. *SAGE Open*, *13*(1). https://doi.org/10.1177/21582440221147022

Materia, E. (2002). Hysterectomy and socioeconomic position in Rome, Italy. *Journal of Epidemiology & Community Health*, *56*(6), 461–465. https://doi.org/10.1136/jech.56.6.461

Mathew, J. L. (2023). Evidence-based medicine: What it is, What it isn't, and Why it is not evidence-biased medicine. *Journal of Medical Evidence*, *4*(2), 170–174. https://doi.org/10.4103/JME.JME_41_23

Mathews, J. J., Chow, R., Wennberg, E., Lau, J., Hannon, B., & Zimmermann, C. (2023). Telehealth palliative care interventions for patients with advanced cancer: A scoping review. *Supportive Care in Cancer*, *31*(8), 451. https://doi.org/10.1007/s00520-023-07907-z

Merrell, R. C. (2015). Geriatric telemedicine: Background and evidence for telemedicine as a way to address the challenges of geriatrics. *Healthcare Informatics Research*, *21*(4), 223–229. https://doi.org/10.4258/hir.2015.21.4.223

Mitchell, D. (2011). Four alternatives to a reductive view of knowledge (seeing with a squint). *Journal of Evaluation in Clinical Practice*, *17*(5), 899–904. https://doi.org/10.1111/j.1365-2753.2011.01724.x

Mohamed, H., Ismail, A., Sutan, R., Rahman, R. A., & Juval, K. (2025). A scoping review of digital technologies in antenatal care: Recent progress and applications of digital technologies. *BMC Pregnancy and Childbirth*, *25*, 153. https://doi.org/10.1186/s12884-025-07209-8

Mol, A. (2002). *The body multiple: Ontology in medical practice*. Duke University Press.

Moreno-Ramírez, D., & Argenziano, G. (2017). Teledermatology and mobile applications in the management of patients with skin lesions. *Acta Dermato Venereologica*, *97*(S218), 31–35. https://doi.org/10.2340/00015555-2718

Newhouse, N., Lupiáñez-Villanueva, F., Codagnone, C., & Atherton, H. (2015). Patient use of email for health care communication purposes across 14 European Countries: An analysis of users according to demographic and health-related factors. *Journal of Medical Internet Research*, *17*(3), e58. https://doi.org/10.2196/jmir.3700

Nordtug, M., Møller, J. E., Matthiesen, S. S., & Brøgger, M. N. (2021). Oralizations in e-mail consultations: A study of general practitioners' use of non-verbal cues in written doctor–patient communication. *Catalan Journal of Communication & Cultural Studies*, *13*(2), 195–211. https://doi.org/10.1386/cjcs_00049_1

Oravainen, T., Airaksinen, M., Hannula, K., & Kvarnström, K. (2021). How physicians renew electronic prescriptions in primary care: Therapeutic decision or technical task?. *International Journal of Environmental Research and Public Health*, *18*(20), 10937. https://doi.org/10.3390/ijerph182010937

Osborne, T. (1994). Anti-medicine and clinical reason 1. In C. Jones & R. Porter (Eds.), *Reassessing foucault: Power, medicine and the body* (pp. 28–48). Routledge.

Payer, L. (1996). *Medicine & culture: Varieties of treatment in the United States, England, West Germany, and France*. Henry Holt and Company.

Porter, R. (1999). *The greatest benefit to mankind: A medical history of humanity from Antiquity to the present*. Fontana Press.

Prodović-Milojković, B., Sinanović, Š., Prodović, T., Milovanović, O., Kilibarda, T., Sretenović, I., Potić, S., Sekulić, J., Bubanj, S., & Subotić-Krivokapić, J. (2024). Digital technologies as support to healthcare systems in promotion of health and prevention of disease: Raising awareness as an aim of communications. *Acta Medica Medianae*, *63*(2), 54–62. https://publisher.medfak.ni.ac.rs/AMM_1/2024/2024-2-broj/celi_radovi/07.Biljana.pdf

Raes, S., Prezzi, A., Willems, R., Heidbuchel, H., & Annemans, L. (2024). Investigating the cost-effectiveness of telemonitoring patients with cardiac implantable electronic devices: Systematic review. *Journal of Medical Internet Research*, *26*, e47616. https://doi.org/10.2196/47616

Rayner, S. (2012). Uncomfortable knowledge: The social construction of ignorance in science and environmental policy discourses. *Economy and Society*, *41*(1), 107–125. https://doi.org/10.1080/03085147.2011.637335

Raz, M. (2024). Uncertain knowledge: The medicalisation of intersex people and the production of ignorance. *Social Sciences*, *13*(8), 385. https://doi.org/10.3390/socsci13080385

Rembrandt. (1632). *The anatomy lesson of Dr. Nicolaes Tulp* [Oil painting]. Wikipedia. https://commons.wikimedia.org/wiki/File:Rembrandt_-_The_Anatomy_Lesson_of_Dr_Nicolaes_Tulp.jpg#/media/File:Rembrandt_-_The_Anatomy_Lesson_of_Dr_Nicolaes_Tulp.jpg

Ritunga, I., Claramita, M., Widaty, S., & Soebono, H. (2024). Challenges and recommendations in the implementation of audiovisual telemedicine communication: A systematic review. *Korean Journal of Medical Education*, *36*(3), 315–326. https://doi.org/10.3946/kjme.2024.305

Rivière, J.-P., Jacob, F., & Girard, A. (2024). Using patient experiences to understand the (missed) digitalisation of the public health service. *Journal of Marketing Management*, *40*(11–12), 968–995. https://doi.org/10.1080/0267257X.2024.2404869

Rose, N. (1994). Medicine, history and the present 1. In C. Jones & R. Porter (Eds.), *Reassessing foucault: Power, medicine and the body* (pp. 48–72). Routledge.

Sendra, A., Torkkola, S., & Parviainen, J. (2023). Non-knowledge in medical practices: Approaching the uses of social media in healthcare from an epistemological perspective. *Journal of Digital Social Research*, *5*(1), 70–89. https://doi.org/10.33621/jdsr.v5i1.152

Serrano, L. P., Maita, K. C., Avila, F. R., Torres-Guzman, R. A., Garcia, J. P., Eldaly, A. S., Haider, C. R., Felton, C. L., Paulson, M. R., Maniaci, M. J., &

Forte, A. J. (2023). Benefits and challenges of remote patient monitoring as perceived by health care practitioners: A systematic review. *The Permanente Journal*, *27*(4), 100–111. https://doi.org/10.7812/TPP/23.022

Song, M., Elson, J., & Bastola, D. (2025). Digital age transformation in patient-physician communication: 25-Year narrative review (1999–2023). *Journal of Medical Internet Research*, *27*, e60512. https://doi.org/10.2196/60512

Sontag, S. (2002). *Illness as metaphor*. Penguin.

Stacey, J. (1997). *Teratologies: A cultural study of cancer*. Routledge.

Strong, P. (1998). The pestilential apocalypse. Modern, postmodern and early modern observations. In R. S. Barbour & G. Huby (Eds.), *Meddling with mythology: AIDS and the social construction of knowledge* (pp. 244–257). Routledge.

Suarez-Lledo, V., & Alvarez-Galvez, J. (2021). Prevalence of health misinformation on social media: Systematic review. *Journal of Medical Internet Research*, *23*(1), e17187. https://doi.org/10.2196/17187

Tariq, A., Aziz, O. A., Arain, F. K., & Munir, M. W. (2021). COVID-19 compels medical practitioners and governments to promote telemedicine practices – a systematic review. *Applied Medical Informatics*, *43*(2), 68–80. https://ami.info.umfcluj.ro/index.php/AMI/article/view/810

Thielmann, R. R. L. C., Hoving, C., Cals, J. W. L., & Crutzen, R. (2023). The effects of online access to general practice medical records perceived by patients: Longitudinal survey study. *Journal of Medical Internet Research*, *25*, e47659. https://doi.org/10.2196/47659

Tokuç, B., & Varol, G. (2023). Medical education in the era of advancing technology. *Balkan Medical Journal*, *40*(6), 395–399. https://doi.org/10.4274/balkanmedj.galenos.2023.2023-7-79

Torkkola, S. (2008). *Sairas juttu: Tutkimus terveysjournalismin teoriasta ja sanomalehden sairaalasta* [Sick story: Research on the theory of health journalism and the newspaper hospital]. Tampere University Press.

Torkkola, S., Tyni, P., Parviainen, J., & Sendra, A. (2024). Terveydenhuollon muuttuvat viestintäkäytännöt: Kyselytutkimus terveydenhuollon asiantuntijoille sosiaalisen median mahdollisuuksista ja uhista potilastyössä [Changing practices in healthcare communication: A survey for healthcare experts about opportunities and threats of social media in patient care]. *Media & Viestintä*, *47*(4), 53–78. https://doi.org/10.23983/mv.130759

Vanhalakka, V., & Ahola, O. (2023, April 23). Matin uusi lonkka [Matti's new hip]. *Aamulehti*. https://www.aamulehti.fi/tampere/art–2000009445720.html

Veerus, P., Lang, K., Toompere, K., & Kirss, F. (2015). Hysterectomy types in Estonia are still different from the Nordic countries. *Acta Obstetricia et Gynecologica Scandinavica*, *94*(5), 489–493. https://doi.org/10.1111/aogs.12614

Vilà, N. (2022, July 18). Lidiar con el cáncer en Afganistán sin oncólogos ni radioterapia [Dealing with cancer in Afghanistan without oncologists or radiation therapy]. *El País*. https://elpais.com/planeta-futuro/2022-07-18/lidiar-con-el-cancer-en-afganistan-sin-oncologos-ni-radioterapia.html

Weiner, J. P. (2012). Doctor–patient communication in the e-health era. *Israel Journal of Health Policy Research*, *1*, 33. https://doi.org/10.1186/2045-4015-1-33

WHO. (2021, February 2). *WHO publishes public health research agenda for managing infodemics*. https://www.who.int/news/item/02-02-2021-who-public-health-research-agenda-for-managing-infodemics

WHO. (2023). *Classification of digital interventions, services and applications in health: A shared language to describe the uses of digital technology for health* (2nd ed.). World Health Organization.

Wilkes, M., Kramer, A., Pugmire, J., Pilkington, C., Zaniello, B., & Zahradka, N. (2024). Hospital is not the home: Lessons from implementing remote technology to support acute inpatient and transitional care in the home in the United States and United Kingdom. *Journal of Medical Internet Research, 26*, e58888. https://doi.org/10.2196/58888

Zadeh, P. E., & Tremblay, M. C. (2016). A review of the literature and proposed classification on e-prescribing: Functions, assimilation stages, benefits, concerns, and risks. *Research in Social and Administrative Pharmacy, 12*(1), 1–19. https://doi.org/10.1016/j.sapharm.2015.03.001

Zhou, Y., Li, S.-J., Huang, R.-Q., Ma, H.-M., Wang, A.-Q., Tang, X.-Y., Pei, R.-Y., & Piao, M.-H. (2024). Behavior change techniques used in self-management interventions based on mHealth apps for adults with hypertension: Systematic review and meta-analysis of randomized controlled trials. *Journal of Medical Internet Research, 26*, e54978. https://doi.org/10.2196/54978

5 Digitalization of sickness

Renegotiating health citizenship

The social dimension of ill health is manifested in sickness. At least theoretically, there are states of being that can be classified as only sick without connection to disease or illness. For example, coercive care can be socially but not medically justified (see, e.g., Høyer, 2000; Tannsjo, 2004). In addition, medical actions have been utilized for political purposes, like the sterilization of women due to disability or ethnicity (Di Giulio, 2024; Mattila, 1999) or the coerced hospitalization of dissidents in totalitarian states (Bonnie, 2002). Sickness, as one of the dimensions of ill health, is also enacted as a social function of medicine. Rudolf Virchow's well-known and used statement from 1848 notes that "medicine is a social science, and politics nothing else but medicine on a large scale" (Mackenbach, 2009; Porter, 1999, p. 643). It summarizes how health promotion and disease reduction depend on the whole society and the political action for changing society (Mackenbach, 2009; Porter, 1999). The medicalization process is both a medical and social process where social problems that are initially not medical become identified as medical problems (see, e.g., Clarke et al., 2003; Conrad, 1992; Zola, 1972). Therefore, medicalization is a process involving medical and social actors but passes over citizens and patients.

Clarke et al. (2003) argue that medicalization transformed into biomedicalization in the 1980s. According to them, biomedicalization involves "the increasingly complex, multisited, multidirectional processes of medicalization, both extended and reconstituted through the new social forms of highly technoscientific biomedicine" (Clarke et al., 2003, p. 161). Unlike in medicalization, in biomedicalization the expansion of power is not based on the expansion of the medical profession but on the expansion of the technoscientific transformations of biomedical organizations, infrastructures, knowledge, and clinical treatments (Clarke et al., 2003). The technoscientific transformation of medicalization seems to relocate citizens and patients and appears to involve them more in the medicalization process. In fact, the increasing use of digital devices and applications for monitoring physical and mental health deepens individuals' biopolitical control of their bodies (Divino, 2024; Köhler et al., 2024). Biomedicalization invites citizens to act as co-producers of medical information, dissolving borders between medicalization objectifying the citizen and

DOI: 10.4324/9781003519607-5

health citizenship demanding active health behaviour. In health citizenship, reconstructed in the digitalization of ill health and healthcare, there are two kinds of activity: the citizens' responsibility to take care of their health and society's responsibility to offer healthcare services to citizens (Jauho & Helén, 2023). In this chapter, we discuss the social dimension of ill health, sickness, and the reconstruction of health citizenship in the digitalization of ill health and healthcare.

Relations between the state, the individual, and the market have been renegotiated in healthcare in recent decades. Health – or the experience of being well – has become an area of personal capital and consumption in an era of constant self-improvement and therapy culture. In this context, the digitalization of sickness has provided people with novel means for optimized health, individual choice, and better access to healthcare services. However, digitalization does not automatically make healthcare more equal or inclusive for all patients (Andreassen et al., 2018; Aronowitz et al., 2021). As Langdridge (2017, p. 1392) reminds us, "the outcomes [of the Internet] are not simply the democratization of medical and health knowledges but something much more complex". Thus, questions such as who has the capabilities and infrastructure to access and provide digital healthcare services or who has the skills to understand the information and data generated by them must be further explored in relation to current performances of health citizenship, in which the right to services for personal well-being implies engaging in proper health behaviour (Mäki-Kuutti, 2020, pp. 46–81).

A recent example of what it means to engage in proper health behaviour can be found in the context of the COVID-19 pandemic. Since the onset of this health crisis, it was expected that citizens maintained good hygiene (e.g., regular handwashing) and physical distance, wore face masks, and consented to vaccinations when required (Sendra et al., 2024). Conversely, citizens who did not engage in these behaviours were punished for it, such as in the form of fines (Sendra et al., 2024). The performances of health citizenship during the COVID-19 pandemic also involved high levels of digitalization, where the provision of remote consultations or the use of mobile apps to detect potential exposures became the norm rather than the exception (Jalabneh et al., 2021; Murphy et al., 2021). In the case of the latter, nevertheless, the effectiveness of this digital technology was not as expected (Hernández-Orallo et al., 2022). Why did individuals not include contact tracing mobile apps in the performances of health citizenship during the COVID-19 pandemic? How did states exercise power through this digital technology, regardless of the evident low levels of adoption?

The answer to these and other questions will guide the discussion related to the digitalization of sickness and the changes around the experience of being ill from the perspective of society. The chapter is divided as follows. First, we will argue what it means to be ill from the perspective of society and how it affects the organization and provision of healthcare. Second, we will describe how patients performed health citizenship before digitalization processes. Third, we will discuss how digitalization is transforming health citizenship into digital health citizenship and outline what it means for the experience of being ill from the perspective of society. The final part of the chapter will deal with emerging tensions related to the digitalization of sickness before presenting the conclusion.

5.1 The experience of being ill from the perspective of society

Sickness involves a top-down approach to the experience of being ill, where institutions and policymakers are the ones determining who can obtain the status of being sick in the eyes of society (Hofmann, 2016). This approach to the experience of being ill has a series of consequences for the social standing of patients, especially in cases where the sickness perspective does not coincide with those of healthcare professionals (disease) and patients (illness). For instance, in conditions where only the illness perspective is present, obtaining the status of being sick in the eyes of society can sometimes be rather challenging – like in the case of fibromyalgia (Paxman, 2021). Likewise, in conditions deemed as sickness but not as disease or illness, this approach to the experience of being ill may lead to discrimination and stigmatization – like in the case of obesity (Hofmann, 2016). As Sánchez-Carracedo (2022, p. 873) explains, patients with this condition often "face a pervasive social stigma based on the typically unproven assumption that their body weight derives primarily from a lack of self-discipline and personal responsibility". We will come back to the case of obesity later in the chapter when discussing how digitalization is transforming health citizenship into digital health citizenship. Moreover, beyond access to support in the form of sick leave or compensation, sickness also decides "whether a person is legally accountable" for their actions (Hofmann, 2016, p. 17). Consequently, implicit to this approach to the experience of being ill is the fact that patients are expected to follow certain norms to be entitled to use healthcare services (Hofmann, 2016; Mäki-Kuutti, 2020, pp. 46–81).

Under the imperative of sickness, patients feel the "moral obligation" of being well by engaging in behaviours that allow them to prevent the experience of being ill (Langdridge, 2017, p. 1392), such as adjusting their diet and changing their lifestyle. These behaviours are sustained on the principles of health promotion, usually driven by top-down approaches, but sometimes also by bottom-up initiatives starting in patient organizations (Rose, 2007). However, the constant evaluation of one's behaviours to meet this moral obligation may generate new problems that contrast with the imperative of sickness, such as patients experiencing problems like anxiety to be (and remain) well (Langdridge, 2017). Therefore, as Lupton (1999, p. 291) argues, "[t]he concept of 'health' is not only located within the body, but also within individual identity, the material and cultural environments, human social relations and policy". In other words, as an individual, one is entitled to use healthcare services not only because one is sick in the eyes of society, but also because one has followed the recommendations made to improve oneself and get back to normal. Likewise, this moral obligation is intertwined with the idea of hope (Novas, 2006), the individual hope of being (and remaining) well if engaging in behaviours that prevent the experience of being ill, embedded with the institutional hope of reducing the burden, economic or otherwise, on healthcare systems (Rose, 2007).

The experience of being ill from the perspective of society (sickness) inevitably affects the organization and provision of healthcare. The process for obtaining a sickness certification, a fundamental step for accessing sick leave benefits, typically starts with a medical consultation with the general practitioner (Tellness, 1989). Over the years, previous research has shown that general practitioners usually support the sick leave requests of patients (Higgins et al., 2014; Hoff et al., 2024), albeit this process is not that straightforward in the absence of disease (Mik-Meyer & Obling, 2012; Wheat et al., 2015). Yet, these requests are often challenged by medical committees, especially in cases of long-term sick leave (Higgins et al., 2014; Nyberg, 2012). Two notions might explain these conflicting views on the sick leave requests of patients. On the one hand, "[s]ickness absence is a complex phenomenon that is influenced strongly by factors other than health" (Whitaker, 2001, p. 422). For example, insurance regulations have a considerable impact on sick leave requests (Söderberg & Alexanderson, 2003), as sick leave represents large economic costs for the state (Nyberg, 2012; Whitaker, 2001). On the other hand, medical committees rely on predetermined guidelines and classifications to approve and renew sick leave requests that do not always align with the experience of being ill from the perspective of the patient (Nyberg, 2012). Recent evidence also indicates that general practitioners are not always comfortable with their role in the process of sickness certification (Hoff et al., 2024), which has been previously criticized for putting "far more weight on the preferences and needs of their patients than [. . .] on the requirements of the organisations that employ their patients" (Higgins et al., 2014, p. 57).

To better understand the mechanisms under which the experience of being ill from the perspective of society (sickness) operates, the case of HIV – and particularly HIV criminalization – is worth discussing. According to a recent report published by UNAIDS (2024, p. 125), up to 156 countries still have in place laws "that criminalize HIV nondisclosure, exposure or transmission explicitly or through general disease laws or prosecutions based on general criminal laws". Some of the countries where HIV criminalization remains explicit include the US and the UK (UNAIDS, 2024). As Hoppe (2014) argues, the case of HIV criminalization shows how a condition is sometimes governed by the law rather than medicine. Through an analysis of 58 court cases of the US state of Michigan, Hoppe (2014, p. 146) shows that narratives describing HIV in relation to death and homicide "are persistent, despite effective therapies that have transformed HIV from a terminal illness to a chronic disease and despite the fact that the vast majority of defendants are not accused of transmitting the virus". One of the reasons behind HIV criminalization is that the law is not up to date with the medical developments regarding this condition (Tatham, 2024; UNAIDS, 2024). Therefore, HIV nondisclosure, exposure, and transmission are socially (rather than medically) controlled in a process that Hoppe (2014) denominates as the criminalization of sickness, where those infected with the virus are punished for not behaving according to the "moral obligation" determined by the law. As UNAIDS (2021) explains, the only thing this criminalization achieves is undermining "effective HIV prevention, treatment, care and support", thus further discriminating against marginalized groups that are already "disproportionately" impacted by HIV criminalization (Hoppe et al., 2022, p. 100).

5.2 Understanding health citizenship

As the introduction to this chapter already hinted at in different ways, the concept of health citizenship is inevitably interlinked with the concept of participation (Harjula, 2016; Komporozos-Athanasiou et al., 2018), particularly the participation of patients, who through various actions directly affect the organization and delivery of healthcare both at the individual and collective levels (Rose, 2007). However, before dissecting the concept of health citizenship and describing how patients performed it before digitalization processes, a definition of the concept itself is necessary. Unfortunately, health citizenship remains poorly defined (Jauho & Helén, 2023). Moreover, most of the literature around health citizenship only focuses on describing what this concept entails. For example, for Groleau (2011, p. 812), health citizenship "involves that health knowledge embodies the illness meaning and experience of patients from the inception of health knowledge to its translation into actions pertaining to clinical communication, health care delivery, as well as public health programs and policy". A further description of what this concept entails is given by Jauho and Helén (2023). For these authors, health citizenship "means that individuals' vital features, capabilities, and potential are used as criteria to assess their membership in a nation or society, to define the quality of their citizenship, and to allow or restrict their access to citizenship entitlements" (Jauho & Helén, 2023, p. 489).

While the latter description touches more on the politicization aspects of the concept (Jauho & Helén, 2023), the former applies more to the biomedicalization dimension of health citizenship (Clarke et al., 2003). However, descriptions of what is known now as health citizenship go back beyond the work of Groleau (2011) and Jauho and Helén (2023). Their and other descriptions of health citizenship are rooted in the notion of biological citizenship (Rose, 2007). According to Rose (2007, p. 132), biological citizenship comprises "all those citizenship projects that have linked their conceptions of citizens to beliefs about the biological existence of human beings". The case of long COVID, discussed in previous chapters (see Chapter 3), serves as one of the most recent examples of biological citizenship and how it is performed. Based on a "biological injury" (Petryna, 2013, p. 36), those affected by long COVID collectively claimed their rights as citizens and eventually managed to be recognized as sick in the eyes of society, thus opening the way to sick leave benefits (e.g., see GOV.UK, n.d.) and access to specialized healthcare services (Savva, 2024). In addition to these collective actions, biological citizenship can also be exercised individually, where the self is evaluated in biological terms and adapts its actions accordingly, mostly in a preventive manner (Rose, 2007). Likewise, the long COVID example shows how this understanding of biological citizenship is reflected in the description of health citizenship by both Groleau (2011) and Jauho and Helén (2023).

Behind this logic of participation, where individuals adopt and change their behaviours to fulfil the "moral obligation" imposed by society, there is also a logic of medical social control (Conrad, 1979; Crawford, 1980). Conrad (1979, p. 1) defines medical social control "as the ways in which medicine functions (wittingly or unwittingly) to secure adherence to social norms". In this context, Conrad (1979) classifies medical social control into medical technology (exercised by medical agents), medical collaboration (exercised by medical agents in collaboration with other authorities), and medical ideology (exercised by medical and non-medical agents alike). For instance, the gatekeeping role of general practitioners in relation to the process of sickness certification is a form of medical collaboration (Conrad, 1979). The aim behind medical social control is to "minimize, eliminate or normalize deviant behavior" (Conrad, 1979, p. 1). A further example of this is the study carried out by Cunningham-Burley et al. (2006), in which the construction of health and sickness was analysed in the context of motherhood and paid work. Cunningham-Burley et al. (2006, p. 404) were able to show that "the assessments of practicalities and perceived possibilities for dealing with adult and child sickness were carried out in the context of making sense of a variety of sometimes contradictory and certainly changing cultural pressures". Not only did the participants in Cunningham-Burley's et al. (2006, p. 401) study report going to work when ill, but they also encouraged their children "not to give in to illness, to carry on and go to school". This once again is a form of medical collaboration in which the participants came up with strategies to fulfil their "moral obligation", minimize the deviant behaviour (i.e., absence from work/school), and avoid being judged as bad mothers/workers (Crawford, 1980).

Prior to the era of digitalization, the options for patients to perform health citizenship were rather limited. The turn towards participatory medicine – and, with it, the turn towards self-care and health promotion – did not start to be obvious until the late 1970s and early 1980s (Crawford, 1980; Killbride & Joffe, 2018), when Western cultures started to take individual responsibility for their health due to "the emergence of a vocal and often aggressive anti-smoking ethic, the proliferation of popular health magazines, and the appearance with amazing frequency of health themes in newspapers, magazines and advertisements for even the most remotely related products" (Crawford, 1980, p. 365). Slowly but steadily, the proliferation of the individual responsibility discourse transformed patients into consumers (Conrad, 2005), commodifying the experience of being ill (Lupton, 2014) and putting the citizen into a state of perpetual risk – that is, "ill but not ill, well but not well" (Langdridge, 2017, p. 1398; Nyberg, 2012). Digitalization not only increased this state of perpetual risk (Felt, 2015) but also opened the avenue for challenging medical social control and engaging in alternative forms of health citizenship (Klausen, 2024), resulting in a connection between empowerment and self-discipline (Henwood & Marent, 2019; Petrakaki et al., 2018, 2021). These and other ways of exercising health citizenship in the digital era will be discussed thoroughly in the following section.

5.3 From health citizenship to digital health citizenship

Health and biological citizenship do not have such a long history like the experience of being ill from the perspective of the patient (illness) and the healthcare professional (disease), albeit "[m]edicine has always performed this social control function" (Crawford, 1980, p. 383). Still, digitalization has allowed the enactment of health and biological citizenship distinctively from when medicine took a participatory turn almost 50 years ago (Table 5.1) – or, at least, it has significantly expanded some of the mechanisms under which the experience of being ill from the perspective of society (sickness) operates (e.g., preventive behaviours). For instance, thanks to digital technologies like apps and platforms, the opportunities for self-care and health promotion are now rather unlimited, to the point that patient-citizens are becoming active agents

Table 5.1 Changes to the experience of being ill from the perspective of society brought by digitalization

Changes	*References*
Digitalization . . .	
. . .is transforming patient-citizens into active agents of medical social control	Conrad (1979), Petersen et al. (2019a)
. . .is leading in some cases to forms of disconnected health citizenship	Bagger et al. (2023), Klausen (2024)
. . .is converting people into preventive patient-citizens	Felt (2015), Langdridge (2017)
. . .is adding layers of complexity to the exercise of patienthood	Fraser et al. (2021), Petersen et al. (2019b), Pols et al. (2019)
. . .is enabling forms of distributed health citizenship	Klausen (2024)

of medical social control (Conrad, 1979) while exercising patienthood in more complicated ways (Fraser et al., 2021). As Petrakaki et al. (2021, Introduction section, para. 2) remind us, "[t]he question of digital technology's influence on health citizenship is prominent for healthcare services in many industrialised countries". The following tries to shed light on the underexplored ways digital health citizenship (Petrakaki et al., 2021) is being exercised, focusing on outlining how digitalization is changing the experience of being ill from the perspective of society.

The first change that digitalization has brought to the experience of being ill from the perspective of society is the transformation of patient-citizens into active agents of medical social control, particularly in the form of medical technology (for a definition of the concept and its typologies, please see the previous section). Medical social control in the form of medical technology was a role previously reserved mostly for healthcare professionals, as only they had "the license and mandate to legally use behavior-controlling drugs and to perform surgery" (Conrad, 1979, p. 7). However, digitalization has created opportunities for other actors (e.g., patient-citizens) to assume this role too (Petersen et al., 2019a). A clear example of this is the case of medications like Ozempic, which patient-citizens are increasingly using off-label to lose weight (Shmerling, 2023). Despite regulations from different administrations, a journalistic investigation found in 2024 that it was "remarkably easy" to purchase compounded versions of Ozempic online (Knibbs, 2024), thus allowing patient-citizens to become active (medical) agents in the medical social control of obesity. In addition to further medicalizing this condition, the adoption of this role by patient-citizens contributed to a shortage of Ozempic and its compounded versions (Shmerling, 2023). While this medication was originally created for treating type 2 diabetes, Ozempic and its compounded versions quickly became a "behaviour-controlling" medication for obesity after going viral on social media thanks to celebrities and influencers (Shmerling, 2023). As Petersen et al. (2019a, p. 489) explain in the case of HIV, the "overwhelming focus on drug treatments [. . .] diverts attention from targeting the social determinants of HIV risk, an approach that could potentially benefit more people overall". This argument is also applicable in the case discussed above, as obesity "is a complex condition influenced by many factors outside an individual's control" (Sánchez-Carracedo, 2022, p. 872).

Another change that digitalization has brought to the experience of being ill from the perspective of society is the possibility of engaging in forms of "disconnected" health citizenship. This type of citizenship does not mean that patient-citizens avoid participating through their actions in the organization and delivery of healthcare altogether, but they rather choose how to engage in health citizenship (Klausen, 2024). Bagger et al. (2023) argue that these behaviours result from the increasing ways of "coerced digital participation" in the organization and delivery of healthcare, where patient-citizens – especially those that live with a chronic illness (Klausen, 2024) – have no other option but to use digital technologies for managing their health. As Klausen (2024, p. 166) explains,

> [b]eing tied up with these infrastructures can be experienced as intrusive, boundary blurring, and associated with intensification of digital labour, and last but not least, experienced as being at odds with personal ideals and wishes for how to live a good life with chronic illness.

In turn, this disconnection perspective might help explain why patient-citizens did not include the use of contact tracing mobile apps in the performance of health citizenship during the COVID-19 pandemic (Hernández-Orallo et al., 2022) and limited their exposure to health and medical information about SARS-CoV-2 as the crisis advanced (Lupton & Lewis, 2021). For patient-citizens, the goal of these and other practices of "disconnected" health citizenship is "to care for themselves" (Klausen, 2024, p. 166) – for example, by "supporting their mental wellbeing" (Lupton & Lewis, 2021, Initial reactions to COVID-19-related information section, para. 6).

These forms of "disconnected" health citizenship might also be related to the next change that digitalization has brought to the experience of being ill from the perspective of society, which is that this digital transformation has exacerbated the number of preventive actions adopted by patient-citizens to comply with the "moral obligation" of being well. That is, in contemporary forms of health citizenship, people have further developed into preventive patient-citizens (Felt, 2015; Langdridge, 2017). As noted by Felt (2015, p. 192), patient-citizens "are actually called on to start to think of themselves as being at risk and as having to engage in preventive practices, with the internet supporting the search for information and feeding such an understanding". However, it is not only the Internet that provides information to the preventive patient-citizen. An autoethnography on the recovery from a heart attack by Langdridge (2017, p. 1395) described how digital technologies like ultrasounds also contribute to the construction of the "subject 'at risk'". While some of these digital technologies remain in the traditional spaces of healthcare (e.g., hospitals), others have permeated spaces previously considered private – what Andreassen et al. (2018) describe as the respatialization of healthcare. This is evident, for instance, in the case of smartwatches. In 2024, there were almost 455 million users of smartwatches worldwide, a significant increase from the almost 98 million users in 2020 (Statista, 2024). Smartwatches are a digital technology that supports the monitoring of different parameters, including heart rate and sleep quality, reporting potential deteriorations in the condition of an individual in the form of notifications (e.g., low heart rate while sleeping) (Triantafyllidis et al., 2024). Therefore, with digitalization, patient-citizens are not only more active in the management of their health, but this role also becomes "more extensive, with people becoming patients well before symptoms appear" (Felt, 2015, p. 192), thus taking the notion of self-care to a whole new level.

Against this background, it is not surprising that another of the changes brought to the experience of being ill from the perspective of society by digitalization is attached to the idea that this digital transformation has complicated the exercising of patienthood for patient-citizens. In a study about young people and sexual health information, Fraser et al. (2021, Conclusions section, para. 1) found that patient-citizens take part in "extensive and complex processes" of information interaction to generate knowledge on sexual health, processes that Petersen et al. (2019b, p. 50) previously denominated as "cartographies of trust" in the context of stem cell treatments. Moreover, these information interaction processes do not rely only on official sources of information (Fraser et al., 2021; Petersen et al., 2019b), as information coming from these sources might be insufficient (Fraser et al., 2021), thus leaving patient-citizens responsible "for seeking and finding the 'truth' even as that truth itself proves relentlessly partial" (Fraser et al., 2021, Conclusions section, para. 2). From this perspective, this requires patient-citizens to have the necessary capabilities (i.e., a determined level of health information literacy) to successfully navigate the information horizon of different conditions, skills that proved to be insufficient, for instance, during the COVID-19 pandemic both for patient-citizens and healthcare professionals alike (Sendra et al., 2023). However, patient-citizens do not only interact with information in the realm of healthcare digitalization, but also with data, which has opened the avenue for different types of the "quantified self" (Lupton, 2016) to arise: (1) those who adopt self-tracking data from a techno-solutionist perspective (the "objectivist-changer" patient-citizen), and (2) those who adopt self-tracking data in a more reflexive manner (the "semiotic-aesthetic" patient-citizen) (Pols et al., 2019). As Pols et al. (2019) explain, the "semiotic-aesthetic" patient-citizen uses self-tracking data to perform "transgressions" – that is, "actions that express resistance to a ritual norm" (Komporozos-Athanasiou et al., 2018, p. 748). Therefore, patient-citizens not only need to learn how to navigate these cartographies of trust (Petersen et al., 2019b), but also ascribe to one of the many roles enabled by digital technologies (Pols et al., 2019).

This last example around self-tracking data brings us to the last change that digitalization has brought to the experience of being ill from the perspective of society, which is that this digital transformation has facilitated forms of "distributed" health citizenship. This concept of "distributed" health citizenship is based on Mol's (2002) idea of distribution. Although Mol's (2002) idea refers to the experience of being ill from the perspective of healthcare professionals (disease), the rationale behind the idea of distribution (i.e., that symptoms of a disease are spread over different places) can also be applied to the experience of being ill from the perspective of society (sickness). With this in mind, by "distributed" health citizenship we mean that healthcare digitalization not only allows the virtual distribution of disease signs but also the virtual distribution of responsibility (Klausen, 2024). That is, patient-citizens are no longer solely responsible for engaging in proper health behaviour, but they share this responsibility with the digital technologies used in the management of their health (Klausen, 2024). This is clearly shown by Klausen (2024, p. 164) in one of the two narrative vignettes presented in her study about disconnective care, where a patient-citizen "needs especially his smart watch to not forget when to take medication". In this context, this and other forms of "distributed" health citizenship raise several questions. For example, what happens when there is a technical fault that prevents the smartwatch from prompting a notification to the patient-citizen? Who would be regarded as "legally accountable" (Hofmann, 2016, p. 17) for not engaging in proper health behaviour, the patient-citizen or the digital technology (and, therefore, the owner behind it)? To answer these and other pressing questions, Klausen (2024, p. 166, emphasis in original) calls for the development of "an ethics of response-ability" that helps us clarify "*which kinds* of data are of use and value and for *who*" amid the increasing digital transformation of the organization and delivery of healthcare.

5.4 Beyond the relationship between empowerment and self-discipline

The previous section has shown the different ways in which digitalization has changed the experience of being ill from the perspective of society, resulting in increasing tensions between empowerment and self-discipline (Henwood & Marent, 2019; Petrakaki et al., 2018, 2021). For example, patients now have more options to challenge the status of being sick in the eyes of society imposed by institutions and policymakers, albeit these practices can be rather demanding (Fraser et al., 2021; Petersen et al., 2019b; Pols et al., 2019), thus forcing patients to "disconnect" from their moral obligation of being well (Bagger et al., 2023; Klausen, 2024) and "distribute" the responsibility for engaging in proper health behaviours (Klausen, 2024) making use of their digital rights as citizens. At the same time, the unlimited opportunities for self-care and health promotion provided by digital technologies are expanding some of the mechanisms under which the experience of being ill from the perspective of society operates, thus placing patients in a state of perpetual risk (Felt, 2015; Langdridge, 2017) to the point that some of them end up assuming roles of medical social control (Conrad, 1979; Petersen et al., 2019a). As Petrakaki et al. (2018, p. 151–152) argue, "this dynamic relationship between empowerment and (self-)discipline [. . .] creates tensions in contemporary healthcare which are manifest in the opportunities for 'health-making' agency". The discussion below intends to reflect on some of these tensions arising from the ways health citizenship is being exercised in the digital era.

The first tension revolves around the idea that, in the digital era, health citizenship is algorithmically produced – at least partially (Petrakaki et al., 2018, 2021). That is, digital health citizenship is "(re)configuring control" (Henwood & Marent, 2019) around the experience of being ill from the perspective of society. For instance, in a study about the cultivation of digital health citizenship, Petrakaki et al. (2021, Discussion section, para. 4) argue that "health apps and platforms encourage patients' towards desirable behaviours" through prompts inserted in the digital technology, such as the reminders to stand up that smartwatches send to users after long periods of seating. Therefore, according to these authors, proper health behaviour does not emanate from the patient, but it is encouraged by the digital technology, which makes them question the "longevity" of this form of health citizenship (Petrakaki et al., 2021, Discussion section, para. 4). Similarly, the status of being sick in the eyes of society can also be algorithmically produced, in this case when using algorithms, for example, to give treatment advice (Petrakaki et al., 2018) or perform diagnostics (Mills & Hilberg, 2019). For instance, through an analysis of an algorithm used to diagnose mental health conditions, Mills and Hilberg (2019, p. 172) were able to demonstrate how the algorithm was created only using quantitative-generated data provided from certain regions, thus generating "a particular imaginary of mental disorder" that systematically excludes knowledge not aligning with these criteria.

Likewise, medical social control is not only reconfigured in the digital era, but institutions and policymakers have new (and significantly more intrusive) options to exercise it. A clear example of these options is the contact tracing mobile apps used during the initial stages of the COVID-19 pandemic (Jalabneh et al., 2021). As Tretter (2023, Nations to Individuals section, para. 9) explains, the benefits of contact tracing mobile apps came at the expense of the "surveillance of the population, invasive intervention [. . .] and, in part, regulation and restriction of their lives". This argument might help explain why contact tracing mobile apps, despite their low levels of effectiveness (Hernández-Orallo et al., 2022), were deployed in many countries – both in the Global North and the Global South – as part of the efforts to curb the effects of the COVID-19 pandemic. On the one hand, contact tracing mobile apps were an opportunity for the state to enlarge the "surveillance apparatus" (Miller et al., 2022, p. 1294) on the population. On the other hand, Rowe (2020, A technology of the self in a neoliberal world section, para. 1) adds that institutions and policymakers strengthened the idea of self-discipline among patient-citizens by making the adoption of contact tracing mobile apps "voluntary rather than compulsory". Altogether, the state found in contact tracing mobile apps a new way to exercise medical social control, where the proper health behaviour (and the moral obligation) was to download this digital technology. The long-term consequences of these and other contemporary mechanisms of medical social control remain unclear, albeit in the case of contact tracing mobile apps, it mainly involves privacy risks (Rowe, 2020). However, what is clear is that "[i]f we want to create this digital future, [. . .] then the rights and responsibilities of the *digital health citizen* of the 21st century need to be established" (Powell et al., 2016, emphasis in original).

A final tension is connected to the notion that, in the digital era, the enactment of health citizenship may result in the generation of resistance to strategies of health promotion control. Once again, the COVID-19 pandemic can help us illustrate this tension. The moment the vaccination started, resistance to vaccination immediately followed, especially after the controversies surrounding the AstraZeneca vaccine were heavily covered in the media (Sendra et al., 2024). This resistance comes from the unlimited possibilities that patient-citizens have at their disposal to participate in the management of their health, including access to information that was previously available only to healthcare professionals (Lupton, 2018). In the case of AstraZeneca, patient-citizens not only had access to information about the vaccine that was previously available only to healthcare professionals but also to its unknowns because of a process that we denominated as the mediatization of ignorance, where these unknowns became mediatized (Sendra et al., 2024). In combination with the ways digital health citizenship is exercised, the mediatization of ignorance most likely "increased the acts of resistance based on unknowns and misinformation toward the biopolitical governance of the COVID-19 pandemic" (Sendra et al., 2024, p. 548). However, resistance does not always come from a combination of the mediatization of ignorance and the ways digital health citizenship is exercised. As Nordtug (2021, p. 1201) found in a study about digital media and HPV vaccination, resistance sometimes comes from a place of not being informed enough, which prompts patient-citizens to get "adequately familiarised with the topic, and not necessarily simply following authority guidelines" before deciding if adopting the health behaviour or not in the name of responsibility.

5.5 Towards a balanced digital health citizenship

The aim of the present chapter was to explore how digitalization has transformed the experience of being ill from the perspective of society (sickness), focusing particularly on analysing the ways in which health citizenship is being renegotiated in the digital era. To do this, we based our discussion on previous research dealing with health citizenship and digital health citizenship from different perspectives, as well as on earlier studies covering the mechanisms under which the experience of being ill operates from the perspective of society.

Under healthcare digitalization, being a good patient-citizen and engaging in proper health behaviour is increasingly determined by the ability of patient-citizens to search, analyse, and use health/medical information and digital healthcare services. One of the more significant findings to emerge from this discussion is that being a patient in the eyes of society is now more complicated (see, e.g., Fraser et al., 2021; Nordtug, 2021), where individuals have at their disposal unlimited options for self-care and health promotion, which in turn increases the pressure to meet the "moral obligation" of being well. To cope with these difficulties, patient-citizens take advantage of these unlimited options to share the responsibility of engaging in proper health behaviour (Klausen, 2024) while at the same time balancing the use of these unlimited options when needed (Bagger et al., 2023; Klausen, 2024). However, it should be noted that being a patient in the eyes of society has become more complicated, also for those less privileged, who, for example, might not have access to the unlimited options for self-care and health promotion provided by digital technologies (Vaagan et al., 2021). In the digital era, these patient-citizens might be denied the right to services for personal well-being simply because they are not meeting the expectations imposed by institutions and policymakers (and possibly also private actors) of being a proper digital patient (Lupton, 2013). As Bagger et al. (2023, Digital resignation and the datafied welfare state section, para. 10) explain, the "datafication of public service and welfare domains introduces new demands on citizens, creates new ambivalences, and opens paths for commercial technology companies". The long-term consequences of this process of datafication need to be further explored, particularly through empirical means.

Overall, the discussion in this chapter strengthens the idea that healthcare digitalization has altered the power relationships between the state, the individual, and the market, opening the route for the digital health citizen (Petrakaki et al., 2021) to emerge. While the state might have more options to exercise medical social control in the digital era, partly thanks to partnerships with the market, the individual also has more power in the enactment of (digital) health citizenship, thus further polarizing the relationship between empowerment and self-discipline (Henwood & Marent, 2019; Petrakaki et al., 2018, 2021). However, the emerging and increasing tensions in the digitalization of the experience of being ill from the perspective of society (sickness) may take this polarization to the point of no return – as happened during the COVID-19 pandemic and the controversies surrounding the AstraZeneca vaccine (Sendra et al., 2024) – thus becoming a risk for the public health of all the population. Therefore, in the digitalization of sickness, it is not only necessary to establish what are the rights and responsibilities of the digital health citizen (Powell et al., 2016) but also to explore how these reconfigured power dynamics between the state, the individual, and the market can become more balanced. As Lie et al. (2022, p. 80–81) argue in a study about people living with chronic conditions and digital healthcare, "[f]or digital healthcare services to promote citizenship, it is imperative that developers and stakeholders understand what specific resources digital healthcare provide in everyday life for citizens with chronic conditions, as well as what the innovations put at stake". We agree with Lie et al. (2022) and extend their plea not only for people living with chronic conditions, but also for all patient-citizens.

References

Andreassen, H. K., Dyb, K., May, C. R., Pope, C. J., & Warth, L. L. (2018). Digitized patient–provider interaction: How does it matter? A qualitative meta-synthesis. *Social Science & Medicine*, *215*, 36–44. https://doi.org/10.1016/j.socscimed.2018.08.036

Aronowitz, S. V., Engel-Rebitzer, E., Dolan, A., Oyekanmi, K., Mandell, D., Meisel, Z., South, E., & Lowenstein, M. (2021). Telehealth for opioid use disorder treatment in low-barrier clinic settings: An exploration of clinician and staff perspectives. *Harm Reduction Journal*, *18*, 119. https://doi.org/10.1186/s12954-021-00572-7

Bagger, C., Einarsson, A. M., Alvarez, V. A., Klausen, M., & Lomborg, S. (2023). Digital resignation and the datafied welfare state. *Big Data & Society*, *10*(2). https://doi.org/10.1177/20539517231206806

Bonnie, R. J. (2002). *Political abuse of psychiatry in the soviet union and in China: Complexities and controversies*. https://doi.org/10.2139/ssrn.1760001

Clarke, A. E., Shim, J. K., Mamo, L., Fosket, J. R., & Fishman, J. R. (2003). Biomedicalization: Technoscientific transformations of health, illness, and U.S. Biomedicine. *American Sociological Review*, *68*(2), 161–194. https://doi.org/10.2307/1519765

Conrad, P. (1979). Types of medical social control. *Sociology of Health & Illness*, *1*(1), 1–11. https://doi.org/10.1111/j.1467-9566.1979.tb00175.x

Conrad, P. (1992). Medicalization and social control. *Annual Review of Sociology*, *18*, 209–232. https://doi.org/10.1146/annurev.so.18.080192.001233

Conrad, P. (2005). The shifting engines of medicalization. *Journal of Health and Social Behavior*, *46*(1), 3–14. https://doi.org/10.1177/002214650504600102

Crawford, R. (1980). Healthism and the medicalization of everyday life. *International Journal of Health Services*, *10*(3), 365–388. https://www.jstor.org/stable/45130677

Cunningham-Burley, S., Backett-Milburn, K., & Kemmer, D. (2006). Constructing health and sickness in the context of motherhood and paid work. *Sociology of Health & Illness*, *28*(4), 385–409. https://doi.org/10.1111/j.1467-9566.2006.00498.x

Di Giulio, M. (2024). Motherhood, mental incompetence, and the denial of reproductive autonomy in the early years of Israeli Statehood. *Journal of Social History*, *57*(4), 550–577. https://doi.org/10.1093/jsh/shad087

Divino, F. (2024). From meditation to techno-mindfulness: On the medicalization of contemplative practices and future prospects. *Histories*, *4*(1), 125–143. https://doi.org/10.3390/histories4010008

Felt, U. (2015). Sociotechnical imaginaries of “the internet,” digital health information and the making of patient-citizens. In S. Hilgartner, C. Miller, & R. Hagendijk (Eds.), *Science and democracy: Making knowledge and making power in the biosciences and beyond* (pp. 176–197). Routledge.

Fraser, S., Moore, D., Waling, A., & Farrugia, A. (2021). Making epistemic citizens: Young people and the search for reliable and credible sexual health information. *Social Science & Medicine*, *276*, 113817. https://doi.org/10.1016/j.socscimed.2021.113817

GOV.UK. (n.d.). *Find help and support if you have long COVID*. https://www.gov.uk/guidance/find-help-and-support-if-you-have-long-covid

Groleau, D. (2011). Embodying “health citizenship” in health knowledge to fight health inequalities. *Revista Brasileira de Enfermagem*, *64*(5), 811–816. https://doi.org/10.1590/s0034-71672011000500002

Harjula, M. (2016). Health citizenship and access to health services: Finland 1900–2000. *Social History of Medicine*, *29*(3), 573–589. https://doi.org/10.1093/shm/hkv144

Henwood, F., & Marent, B. (2019). Understanding digital health: Productive tensions at the intersection of sociology of health and science and technology studies. *Sociology of Health & Illness*, *41*(S1), 1–15. https://doi.org/10.1111/1467-9566.12898

Hernández-Orallo, E., Manzoni, P., Calafate, C. T., & Cano, J. (2022). A methodology for evaluating digital contact tracing apps based on the COVID-19 experience. *Scientific Reports*, *12*, 12728. https://doi.org/10.1038/s41598-022-17024-2

Higgins, A., Porter, S., & O'Halloran, P. (2014). General practitioners' management of the long-term sick role. *Social Science & Medicine*, *107*, 52–60. https://doi.org/10.1016/j.socscimed.2014.01.044

Hoff, E. H., Kraft, K. B., Moe, C. F., Nylenna, M., Østby, K. A., & Mykletun, A. (2024). The cost of saying no: General practitioners' gatekeeping role in sickness absence certification. *BMC Public Health*, *24*, 439. https://doi.org/10.1186/s12889-024-17993-1

Hofmann, B. (2016). Disease, Illness, and Sickness. In M. Solomon, J. R. Simon, & H. Kincaid (Eds.), *The Routledge companion to philosophy of medicine* (pp. 16–26). Routledge.

Hoppe, T. (2014). From sickness to badness: The criminalization of HIV in Michigan. *Social Science & Medicine*, *101*, 139–147. https://doi.org/10.1016/j.socscimed.2013.11.007

Hoppe, T., McClelland, A., & Pass, K. (2022). Beyond criminalization: Reconsidering HIV criminalization in an era of reform. *Current Opinion in HIV and AIDS*, *17*(2), 100–105. https://doi.org/10.1097/COH.0000000000000715

Høyer, G. (2000). On the justification for civil commitment. *Acta Psychiatrica Scandinavica*, *101*(399), 65–71. https://doi.org/10.1111/j.0902-4441.2000.007s020[dash]16.x

Jalabneh, R., Syed, H. Z., Pillai, S., Apu, E. H., Hussein, M. R., Kabir, R., Arafat, S. M. Y., Majumder, A. A., & Saxena, S. K. (2021). Use of mobile phone apps for contact tracing to control the COVID-19 pandemic: A literature review. In S. N. Mohanty, S. K. Saxena, S. Satpathy, & J. M. Chatterjee (Eds.), *Applications of artificial intelligence in COVID-19* (pp. 389–404). Springer.

Jauho, M., & Helén, I. (2023). Citizenship by vitality: Rethinking the concept of health citizenship. *Distinktion: Journal of Social Theory*, *24*(3), 467–487. https://doi.org/10.1080/1600910X.2022.2057561

Killbride, M. K., & Joffe, S. (2018). The new age of patient autonomy: Implications for the patient-physician relationship. *JAMA*, *320*(19), 1973–1974. https://doi.org/10.1001/jama.2018.14382

Klausen, M. (2024). Disconnective care: Chronic illness and digital patienthood. In K. Albris, K. Fast, F. Karlsen, A. Kaun, S. Lomborg, & T. Syvertsen (Eds.), *The digital backlash and the paradoxes of disconnection* (pp. 153–170). Nordicom. https://doi.org/10.48335/9789188855961-8

Knibbs, K. (2024, July 12). It's shockingly easy to buy off-brand ozempic online, even if you don't need it. *Wired*. https://www.wired.com/story/

glp1-ozempic-wegovy-semaglutide-compounding-pharmacies-hims-reflexmd-alan-meds-henry-ro-getthinmd/

Köhler, C., Bartschke, A., Fürstenau, D., Schaaf, T., & Salgado-Baez, E. (2024). The value of smartwatches in the health care sector for monitoring, nudging, and predicting: Viewpoint on 25 years of research. *Journal of Medical Internet Research*, *26*, e58936. https://doi.org/10.2196/58936

Komporozos-Athanasiou, A., Fudge, N., Adams, M., & McKevitt, C. (2018). Citizen participation as political ritual: Towards a sociological theorizing of 'health citizenship'. *Sociology*, *52*(4), 744–761. https://doi.org/10.1177/0038038516664683

Langdridge, D. (2017). Recovery from heart attack, biomedicalization, and the production of a contingent health citizenship. *Qualitative Health Research*, *27*(9), 1391–1401. https://doi.org/10.1177/1049732316668818

Lie, S. S., Fjetland, K. J., & Tokovska, M. (2022). How may digital healthcare influence citizenship for people with chronic conditions? A narrative review. In K. J. Fjetland, A. Gjermestad, & I. M. Lid (Eds.), *Lived citizenship for persons in vulnerable life situations: Theories and practices* (pp. 79–95). Scandinavian University Press. https://doi.org/10.18261/9788215053790-2022-05

Lupton, D. (1999). 'Developing the "whole me"': Citizenship, neoliberalism and the contemporary health and physical education curriculum. *Critical Public Health*, *9*(4), 287–300. https://doi.org/10.1080/09581599908402941

Lupton, D. (2013). The digitally engaged patient: Self-monitoring and self-care in the digital health era. *Social Theory & Health*, *11*(3), 256–270. https://doi.org/10.1057/sth.2013.10

Lupton, D. (2014). The commodification of patient opinion: The digital patient experience economy in the age of big data. *Sociology of Health & Illness*, *36*(6), 856–869. https://doi.org/10.1111/1467-9566.12109

Lupton, D. (2016). *The quantified self: A sociology of self-tracking*. Polity Press.

Lupton, D. (2018). *Digital health: Critical and cross-disciplinary perspectives*. Routledge.

Lupton, D., & Lewis, S. (2021). Learning about COVID-19: A qualitative interview study of Australians' use of information sources. *BMC Public Health*, *21*(1), 662. https://doi.org/10.1186/s12889-021-10743-7

Mackenbach, J. P. (2009). Politics is nothing but medicine at a larger scale: Reflections on public health's biggest idea. *Journal of Epidemiology & Community Health*, *63*(3), 181–184. https://doi.org/10.1136/jech.2008.077032

Mäki-Kuutti, A. M. (2020). *Terveyskuri mediayhteiskunnassa: Populaari terveysviestintä toimijuuden ja hallinnan kenttänä* [Health discipline in media society. Popular health communication as a field of agency and governmentality]. [Doctoral dissertation, Tampere University]. Trepo.

Mattila, M. (1999). *Kansamme parhaaksi: Rotuhygienia Suomessa vuoden 1935 sterilointilakiin asti* [In Our Nation's Best Interest: Eugenics in Finland until the promulgation of the Sterilization Law of 1935]. Suomen Historiallinen Seura.

Mik-Meyer, N., & Obling, A. R. (2012). The negotiation of the sick role: General practitioners' classification of patients with medically unexplained symptoms. *Sociology of Health & Illness*, *34*(7), 1025–1038. https://doi.org/10.1111/j.1467-9566.2011.01448.x

Miller, J. P., Sander, A., & Srinivasan, S. (2022). Control, extract, legitimate: COVID-19 and digital techno-opportunism across Africa. *Development and Change*, *53*(6), 1283–1307. https://doi.org/10.1111/dech.12734

Mills, C., & Hilberg, E. (2019). 'Built for expansion': The 'social life' of the WHO's mental health GAP intervention guide. *Sociology of Health & Illness*, *41*(S1), 162–175. https://doi.org/10.1111/1467-9566.12870

Mol, A. (2002). *The body multiple: Ontology in medical practice*. Duke University Press.

Murphy, M., Scott, L. J., Salisbury, C., Turner, A., Scott, A., Denholm, R., Lewis, R., Iyer, G., Macleod, J., & Horwood, J. (2021). Implementation of remote consulting in UK primary care following the COVID-19 pandemic: A mixed-methods longitudinal study. *British Journal of General Practice*, *71*(704), e166–e177. https://doi.org/10.3399/BJGP.2020.0948

Nordtug, M. (2021). Who knows best? Health risks and digital media engagement in discourses relating to human papillomavirus vaccination. *Sociology of Health & Illness*, *43*(5), 1191–1205. https://doi.org/10.1111/1467-9566.13284

Novas, C. (2006). The political economy of hope: Patients' organizations, science and biovalue. *BioSocieties*, *1*(3), 289–305. https://doi.org/10.1017/S1745855206003024

Nyberg, D. (2012). 'You need to be healthy to be Ill': Constructing sickness and framing the body in Swedish healthcare. *Organization Studies*, *33*(12), 1671–1692. https://doi.org/10.1177/0170840612457615

Paxman, C. G. (2021). "Everyone thinks I am just lazy": Legitimacy narratives of Americans suffering from fibromyalgia. *Health: An Interdisciplinary Journal for the Social Study of Health, Illness and Medicine*, *25*(1), 121–137. https://doi.org/10.1177/1363459319857457

Petersen, A., Schermuly, A. C., & Anderson, A. (2019a). The shifting politics of patient activism: From bio-sociality to bio-digital citizenship. *Health*, *23*(4), 478–494. https://doi.org/10.1177/1363459318815944

Petersen, A., Tanner, C., & Munsie, M. (2019b). Navigating the cartographies of trust: How patients and carers establish the credibility of online treatment claims. *Sociology of Health & Illness*, *41*(S1), 50–64. https://doi.org/10.1111/1467-9566.12872

Petrakaki, D., Hilberg, E., & Waring, J. (2018). Between empowerment and self-discipline: Governing patients' conduct through technological self-care. *Social Science & Medicine*, *213*, 146–153. https://doi.org/10.1016/j.socscimed.2018.07.043

Petrakaki, D., Hillberg, E., & Waring, J. (2021). The cultivation of digital health citizenship. *Social Science & Medicine*, *270*, 113675. https://doi.org/10.1016/j.socscimed.2021.113675

Petryna, A. (2013). *Life exposed: Biological citizens after chernobyl*. Princeton University Press.

Pols, J., Willems, D., & Aanestad, M. (2019). Making sense with numbers. Unravelling ethico-psychological subjects in practices of self-quantification. *Sociology of Health & Illness*, *41*(S1), 98–115. https://doi.org/10.1111/1467-9566.12894

Porter, R. (1999). *The greatest benefit to mankind: A medical history of humanity from Antiquity to the present*. Fontana Press.

Powell, J., Newhouse, N., Boylan, A., & Williams, V. (2016). Digital health citizens and the future of the NHS. *Digital Health*, *2*. https://doi.org/10.1177/2055207616672033

Rose, N. (2007). *The politics of life itself: Biomedicine, power, and subjectivity in the Twenty-First Century*. Princeton University Press.

Rowe, F. (2020). Contact tracing apps and values dilemmas: A privacy paradox in a neo-liberal world. *International Journal of Information Management*, *55*, 102178. https://doi.org/10.1016/j.ijinfomgt.2020.102178

Sánchez-Carracedo, D. (2022). Obesity stigma and its impact on health: A narrative review. *Endocrinología, Diabetes y Nutrición*, *69*(10), 868–877. https://doi.org/10.1016/j.endien.2021.12.007

Savva, A. (2024, February 7). Long Covid sufferers express relief at specialist help. *BBC*. https://www.bbc.com/news/articles/cgrl05ydedlo

Sendra, A., Torkkola, S., & Parviainen, J. (2023). Non-knowledge in medical practices: Approaching the uses of social media in healthcare from an epistemological perspective. *Journal of Digital Social Research*, *5*(1), 70–89. https://doi.org/10.33621/jdsr.v5i1.152

Sendra, A., Torkkola, S., & Parviainen, J. (2024). AstraZeneca vaccine controversies in the media: Theorizing about the mediatization of ignorance in the context of the COVID-19 vaccination campaign. *Health Communication*, *39*(3), 541–551. https://doi.org/10.1080/10410236.2023.2171951

Shmerling, R. H. (2023, February 21). What happens when a drug goes viral?. *Harvard Health Publishing*. https://www.health.harvard.edu/blog/what-happens-when-a-drug-goes-viral-2023022128920

Söderberg, E., & Alexanderson, K. (2003). Sickness certification practices of physicians: A review of the literature. *Scandinavian Journal of Public Health*, *31*(6), 460–474. https://www.jstor.org/stable/45138014

Statista. (2024, September 1). *Smartwatches*. https://www.statista.com/outlook/hmo/digital-health/digital-fitness-well-being/fitness-trackers/smartwatches/worldwide

Tannsjo, T. (2004). The convention on human rights and biomedicine and the use of coercion in psychiatry. *Journal of Medical Ethics*, *30*(5), 430–434. https://doi.org/10.1136/jme.2002.000703

Tatham, C. (2024). Life and love under criminalization: The experiences of people living with HIV in Canada. *PLoS One*, *19*(7), e0306894. https://doi.org/10.1371/journal.pone.0306894

Tellness, G. (1989). Sickness certification in general practice: A review. *Family Practice*, *6*(1), 58–65. https://doi.org/10.1093/fampra/6.1.58

Tretter, M. (2023). Sovereignty in digital and contact tracing apps. *Digital Society*, *2*, 2. https://doi.org/10.1007/s44206-022-00030-2

Triantafyllidis, A., Kondylakis, H., Katehakis, D., Kouroubali, A., Alexiadis, A., Segkouli, S., Votis, K., & Tzovaras, D. (2024). Smartwatch interventions in healthcare: A systematic review of the literature. *International Journal of Medical Informatics*, *190*, 105560. https://doi.org/10.1016/j.ijmedinf.2024.105560

UNAIDS. (2021). *HIV criminalization*. https://www.unaids.org/sites/default/files/media_asset/01-hiv-human-rights-factsheet-criminalization_en.pdf

UNAIDS. (2024). *The urgency of now: AIDS at a crossroads*. https://www.unaids.org/sites/default/files/media_asset/2024-unaids-global-aids-update_en.pdf

Vaagan, R. W., Torkkola, S., Sendra, A., Farré, J., & Lovari, A. (2021). A critical analysis of the digitization of healthcare communication in the EU: A comparison of Italy, Finland, Norway, and Spain. *International Journal of Communication*, *15*, 1718–1740. https://ijoc.org/index.php/ijoc/article/view/15399

Wheat, H. C., Barnes, R. K., & Byng, R. (2015). Practices used for recommending sickness certification by general practitioners: A conversation analytic study of UK primary care consultations. *Social Science & Medicine*, *126*, 48–58. https://doi.org/10.1016/j.socscimed.2014.12.006

Whitaker, S. C. (2001). The management of sickness absence. *Occupational & Environmental Medicine*, *58*(6), 420–424. https://doi.org/10.1136/oem.58.6.420

Zola, I. K. (1972). Medicine as an institution of social control. *The Sociological Review*, *20*(4), 487–504. https://doi.org/10.1111/j.1467-954X.1972.tb00220.x

6 Patienthood and healthcare communication in the digital era

The previous chapters have discussed how the digitalization of healthcare has respatialized and retemporalized ill health and care. These changes are manifested in the interactions between care providers and care receivers but also in healthcare communication more generally. Furthermore, we have seen large-scale, promising opportunities to improve the delivery of healthcare services, access to health and medical information by citizens and patients, participation in care decision-making, and the empowerment of patients. However, besides these advantages, there are plenty of doubts concerning digitalization itself and the challenges driven by the virtualization of healthcare and the interaction between the care provider and care receiver. Usually, the evaluation of digital services focuses on two topics: (1) use and assessment of digital public services by citizens and (2) the impact of the digital transformation on the relationship between citizens and public authorities (Jæger, 2021). In the context of the digitalization of healthcare, we call the use and assessment of digital public services by citizens "infrastructural factors", which include both the technical conditions – like the availability of Internet or devices for using digital healthcare services – and digital literacy – i.e., the ability to use digital healthcare services. For the impact of the digital transformation on the relationship between citizens and public authorities, we use the term "interactional factors", which facilitates online communication between healthcare service providers and receivers. These interactional factors include online communication skills and software, applications, and platforms offering virtual places for communication.

Infrastructural factors are essential factors for enacting digital citizenship. Participation in online society requires regular access to and the effective use of information and communication technologies (Mossberger, 2008; Mossberger et al., 2007, pp. 6–15). At the individual level, digital citizenship requires both having easy access to the Internet for daily use and the technical skills and educational competence to find and use information and communicate with others online (Mossberger, 2008; Mossberger et al., 2007, pp. 6–15). In the context of the digitalization of healthcare, evidence indicates that the infrastructural factors needed for accessing and using digital healthcare services are not equally

DOI: 10.4324/9781003519607-6

available for all citizens (Stephens & Mankee-Williams, 2021). Particularly, Mandi Stephens and Anna Mankee-Williams (2021, p. 57) point out that "individuals from lower income households, individuals residing in areas with poor digital infrastructure, and individuals without adequate digital skills are at risk of being excluded from digital healthcare". However, the findings of previous studies on the relationship between socio-demographic profiles and the use of digital technologies differ. On the one hand, some studies show that individuals with good socioeconomic conditions, high educational levels, and a young age are more likely to use digital technologies, the Internet, and social media (Yildiz Durak & Seferoğlu, 2020). On the other hand, a German study conducted by Anja Knöchelmann et al. (2024) demonstrated that active users of digital healthcare services are those with the lowest level of education. Furthermore, older people were identified in the study as both active users of digital healthcare services and users who reject them (Knöchelmann et al., 2024).

Besides the technical conditions to use digital services related to infrastructural factors, there are also immaterial factors manifesting in digital literacy – i.e., the ability to use digital services. According to classical definitions, digital literacy is the competence to write, read, and deal with information as well as use different digital technologies (Njenga, 2018). However, the current understanding of digital literacy is more diverse, where digital literacy is understood not only as one literacy but as multiple literacies covering "both the mastery of information and communication technology skills and generic and critical skills required to engage in social practices across boundaries of culture, institutions, countries and territories" (Njenga, 2018, p. 2). These immaterial infrastructural factors of digital citizenship are in harmony with digital health citizenship, which is heavily rooted in health literacy. The WHO (2021, p. 6) defines health literacy as

> the personal knowledge and competencies that accumulate through daily activities, social interactions and across generations. Personal knowledge and competencies are mediated by the organizational structures and availability of resources that enable people to access, understand, appraise and use information and services in ways that promote and maintain good health and well-being for themselves and those around them.

Compared to this definition of health literacy, digital health literacy requires both competence to find, understand, and use health and medical information and competence to search, evaluate, and appraise health and medical information spreading out on the Internet and social media. In the context of the digitalization of healthcare, the big question is whether healthcare organizations are responsible for providing education on digital health literacy or if this educational task belongs to other organizations. Although healthcare organizations are not asked to educate citizens and patients in (digital) health literacy, in the digitalization of healthcare communication, it is necessary to take into consideration the multiple literacies behind digital health literacy. This especially concerns all communicative actions that healthcare communication consists of, starting with the interactions between care providers and care receivers up to the delivery and use of medical information and the patients' own health records.

The impact of the digital transformation on the relationship between citizens and public authorities – i.e., the interactional factors – is based on online communication. Findings from a study reviewing digital citizenship in the academic literature by Birgit Jæger (2021) demonstrate dramatic changes in the nature of professionals' relationship with citizens in the era of digital communication. In particular, these changes may weaken the position of vulnerable citizens (Jæger, 2021; see also Buchert et al., 2024). As we have discussed in the previous chapters, a more informed patient has a greater ability to participate in care decision-making, manifested in the interactions between care providers and care receivers. When digitalization strengthens patients' access to health and medical information and the patients' own medical records, this also promotes digital health citizenship.

However, digitalization does not automatically result in improved health citizenship. In spite of all the benefits of digitalization, engagement with digital healthcare services can be experienced as coercive (Bagger et al., 2023; Rousaki et al., 2024) and exacerbate feelings of exclusion (Rousaki et al., 2024). For example, evidence indicates that home monitoring for old people based on telecare can be a coercive action that does not recognize individual daily practices (Mort et al., 2013). Another study found that "people who are experiencing disadvantaged circumstances in their everyday lives face insurmountable hurdles" in using digital services, including those related to healthcare (Buchert et al., 2024, p. 947). If motivation for the digitalization of healthcare services is driven by the difficult financial climate and the demand for cost savings in healthcare, this may lead to ignoring the users' experiences and needs (Eden & Bloor, 2010; Mort et al., 2013). Daniel Eden and Jonathan Bloor (2010, p. 121) pointed out already in 2010 that "investment in information technology should emphasise the long-term advantages for patients rather than short-term financial savings".

To improve the experience of citizens and patients with digital healthcare services, including alleviating these feelings of coercion and exclusion, the communicative tasks that drive the digital transformation of healthcare must be recognized and brought to the forefront. And not only do these communicative tasks have to take centre stage, but they must also be investigated from different perspectives. As we have seen throughout this book, digital healthcare services should be evaluated on the basis of how they support these communicative tasks, as "[a]n essential premise of maintaining good health is to manage health information" (Eriksson-Backa et al., 2022, p. 314). This can be done by adopting an information studies perspective to the study of healthcare digitalization (Järvelin et al., 2015). For example, by adopting a task-based approach (Järvelin et al., 2015, p. 24), digital healthcare services – understood here as information retrieval systems – "are not evaluated as stand-alone systems but rather as components in interaction with associated human behaviors and factors".

Likewise, digital healthcare services should also be analysed in terms of how they change the ways these communicative tasks are performed, as "[t]he widespread use of digital technology has changed the mode of interpersonal interaction and the construction of social relationships" (Zhao & Wang, 2023, Social relationships and interactions section, para. 1). This can be done by adopting a sociological perspective to the study of healthcare digitalization (Zhao & Wang, 2023). Furthermore, digital healthcare services should be investigated for how they impact the order of knowledge through the execution of these communicative tasks, as "[d]igital media tend to destabilize the traditional knowledge order" (Neuberger et al., 2023, p. 180). This can be done by adopting an epistemological perspective to the study of healthcare digitalization (Neuberger et al., 2023). As a sub-field of health communication (see Chapter 1), healthcare communication is as multifaceted as health communication (Torkkola, 2016); thus, it should be explored and theorized as such.

6.1 Digitalization of communicative tasks

Throughout this book, we have shown how healthcare digitalization has led to the respatialization and retemporalization of care and reconstructed relations in healthcare, particularly the interactions between care providers and care receivers. Following these changes, the tasks in healthcare have also been altered. There are not only new tasks driven by technology; systems for digital communication imply more invisible work for both care providers and care receivers, and lead to the reallocation of care work that demands patients be responsible for their care at home (Andreassen et al., 2018). The digitalization of patient-provider interaction leads to altered interaction chains in healthcare, affecting structures of participation, power, and influence that alter not only the relationship between the care provider and the care receiver but also reconstruct ill health (see Andreassen et al., 2018).

In the digitalization of healthcare communication, there are plenty of changes that demand the reorientation of individual healthcare professionals and the organization responsible for the communication environment. More concretely, the digitalization of healthcare communication requires the reallocation of communicative tasks. In Table 6.1, we have collected the digital changes to healthcare services and the communication responses needed to realize these changes.

Although healthcare organizations do not carry general responsibility for health and medical information delivery, in reality, this information cannot be ignored. Rather, both healthcare organizations and healthcare professionals need to pay more attention not only to the quality of the information but also to

Table 6.1 Communicative tasks in the digitalization of healthcare

Digital functions of healthcare	*Most typical communicative tasks for healthcare professionals*
Health/medical information delivery (including dis- and misinformation)	- Produce and deliver health and medical information by healthcare organizations in digital form - Follow health and medical information delivery generally - Recognize experiential knowledge of care receivers delivered in digital form - Recognize medical knowledge produced by care receivers delivered in digital form - Recognize online dis- and misinformation - Facilitate care receivers' digital health literacy (especially health information literacy)
Digital patient records	- Facilitate care providers' and care receivers' access to records - Facilitate care receivers' digital health literacy (especially medical literacy) - Ensure data protection - Facilitate data users' ability to handle information securely - Recognize the possibility of co-writing by care receivers
Digital medical and nursing consultations and remote monitoring	- Facilitate and develop technical solutions to improve online communication - Recognize and understand the communicative limitations of virtual healthcare - Arrange further education in online communication for care providers - Arrange service guidance for care receivers
Digital platforms (e.g., social media) for the care receiver	- Facilitate secure environments for the discussion and exchange of experiential knowledge - Facilitate secure environments for receiving and providing peer support - Follow health topics in discussions - Search for weak signals on patient safety or other challenges in healthcare services - Facilitate care providers' participation in digital platforms and social media - Cooperate with service administrations on health and medical information delivery
Digital platforms for the care provider	- Facilitate the use of health and medical information with or without AI - Facilitate consultation between care providers in secure environments - Offer training in communication skills

how citizens and patients use it. The enormous information flow of health and medical topics is impossible to follow extensively, as is trying to completely control it and its impact on citizens' health behaviours and the use of healthcare services. Although there are grounded doubts about the impact of health communication campaigns on health behaviour (Torkkola, 2016), we cannot say that the media, social media, or the health and medical information delivered through the Internet has no impact on citizens' health knowledge, attitudes, or behaviour. Recent studies have shown, for example, that social networks can generate, accelerate, or maintain health behaviour (Hunter et al., 2019). Likewise, social media played a significant role globally in promoting preventive behaviours during the COVID-19 pandemic (Talie Fenta et al., 2024).

In addition to the positive impacts of new media on health, evidence also indicates plenty of negative impacts, especially in relation to the online spread of health dis- and misinformation (see, e.g., Do Nascimento et al., 2022; Heley et al., 2025). Misinformation has become a societal and systemic issue that needs significant resources to be resolved – if this is even possible (Dickinson et al., 2025). Thus, healthcare organizations are facing complex problems that are difficult or even impossible to control. A possible way out is to increase our understanding of the online information environment and adapt the communicative actions to this new communication landscape. In the context of the digitalization of healthcare, to increase our understanding of virtual healthcare and medical information, it is imperative that healthcare organizations and healthcare professionals know what kind of health and medical information is spreading virtually and how it is discussed among laypeople. Therefore, the traditional, one-way, and authoritarian communication model of healthcare does not work anymore, and external communication cannot be allocated only to communication professionals. In the future, healthcare professionals will probably need to be more involved with external communication. As a result, changes in professional responsibility and education, as well as the further education of healthcare experts, will be necessary. Moreover, these changes will also result in a redivision of labour in healthcare organizations.

Unlike general health and medical information, patient records are more controlled by healthcare organizations. Although health literacy does not directly belong to the responsibilities of healthcare authorities, the providers of healthcare services have a lot of opportunities to support the patients' ability to understand medical texts – and, therefore, facilitate patient empowerment. One solution for making impenetrable medical language more understandable involves implementing and using simplified language in healthcare – e.g., Easy Language (Valkendorff & Vanhatalo, 2025). Most likely, this solution could work in online environments too, but the digital realm can also offer novel solutions for opening medical language to laypeople, including medical dictionaries, Q&A services, and perhaps AI assistance. In this case, healthcare professionals also need to be more involved in these new communicative tasks, as they cannot be handled by communication experts only.

Likewise, digital medical and nursing consultations and remote monitoring are not only technical solutions; they also reconstruct communicative relations (see, e.g., Marent & Henwood, 2023). To understand telemedicine (and virtual healthcare in general), we need to go beyond techno-centric approaches and explore how the respatialization and retemporalization of care are manifested in the interactions and power relations between care providers and care receivers. As we have seen throughout this book, more informed patients can be more empowered, have more ability to participate in care decision-making, and have even more opportunities to challenge medical authority and promote their own choices, demanding reorientation from doctors and other healthcare professionals. These reconstructed interactions between care providers and care receivers can be more challenging in online environments. Therefore, further education on online communication is required both from healthcare organizations and medical education providers.

However, we must also not lose sight of the fact that not all patients use or accept digital opportunities for healthcare services. From the viewpoint of the patients' independence, coercive digitalization is not a solution, and healthcare organizations must have alternative forms of communication in addition to the virtual ones, albeit these alternative ways of communication might face criticism due to the extra costs and increased workload for healthcare organizations and healthcare professionals. In this context, a debate on the right to paper documentation is highly likely to happen in the future. Because of these parallel functions needed in the transition towards totally digital healthcare communication, the coming years are going to be very challenging for healthcare organizations, and the promises to improve healthcare expenditure associated with the digitalization of healthcare are not going to be totally fulfilled due to these duplicate costs.

6.2 Digitalization of patienthood

Throughout this book, we have also discussed how the digitalization of healthcare communication is altering patienthood. Patienthood as a sociocultural construction invites the ill person to be a patient in certain conditions that are rooted in the dimensions of ill health – i.e., illness, disease, and sickness.

In the digitalization of illness, patienthood results in enhanced activism, the co-construction of health knowledge, and the co-production of science communication thanks to increased access to health and medical information and opportunities for peer support, generating new disease regimes where the experience of being ill from the perspective of the patient takes a more relevant role. In the digitalization of disease, both sides of medicine – science (medical knowledge) and art (medical practice) – are transformed by the digitalization of healthcare. On the one hand, (digital) medical knowledge has enabled the rise of a more informed patient. As a result, doctor-patient interactions have improved, but conflicts have also been generated due to challenges to the authority of healthcare professionals. On the other hand, in (digital) medical practices, signs – i.e., symptoms – of disease carried by the patient have spread out in the digital realm. Consequently, in virtual medicine, the patient does not always need to carry the symptoms of a disease to be inspected by the medical gaze. In the digitalization of sickness – i.e., the social response to illness – patienthood and citizenship unite into (digital) health citizenship, where the ways that an ill person is a good patient-citizen and engages in proper health behaviours are increasingly determined by the ability to search for, analyse, and use both digital healthcare services and health/medical information, where the ill person ends up regulating the participation in the organization and delivery of healthcare and sharing the responsibility for care with digital healthcare services.

The digitalization of ill health results in two conflicting consequences for patienthood. As we have seen throughout this book, the digitalization of ill health and healthcare services can both facilitate and weaken the empowerment of patients. Firstly, virtual medicine cuts both the disease and the patient carrying it into pieces and spreads them out into the digital realm, thus making it difficult to say where the patient is located. A disease can be diagnosed, and a patient can be treated without consultation between the doctor and the patient. This can be understood as the end of the patient driven by the birth of modern medicine. Secondly, digital healthcare services – like the delivery of health and medical information and easier access to personal health records and peer support – as well as the demands and opportunities for personal health promotion, reconstruct a patienthood that is now more active and a health citizenship that has new duties and rights.

The reconstruction of patienthood becomes even more complex under the digitalization of healthcare communication (see Figure 6.1). In the digital era, the communication environment of healthcare communication (see Figure 1.1) has changed, but the digital functions of healthcare have not replaced the previous communicative relations. Instead, the digital functions of healthcare are working with and between communication actors inside and outside healthcare. Consequently, the communicative relationship between healthcare and other organizations may become complicated. For example, during the COVID-19 pandemic, hesitance surrounding the AstraZeneca vaccine was more based on the impact of the negative discussions taking place on social media rather than on the medical facts communicated by health authorities (Sendra et al., 2024).

Therefore, healthcare organizations and healthcare professionals are facing an altered communication environment not only within internal communication but also within external communication, which, due to multiplying communication platforms and channels, demands more attention from healthcare organizations and healthcare professionals. The topics that used to be seen and treated as internal matters of the organization can now be challenged by "outsiders", thus requiring the organization or individual professional to participate in public discussion. As previously described, these new communicative tasks

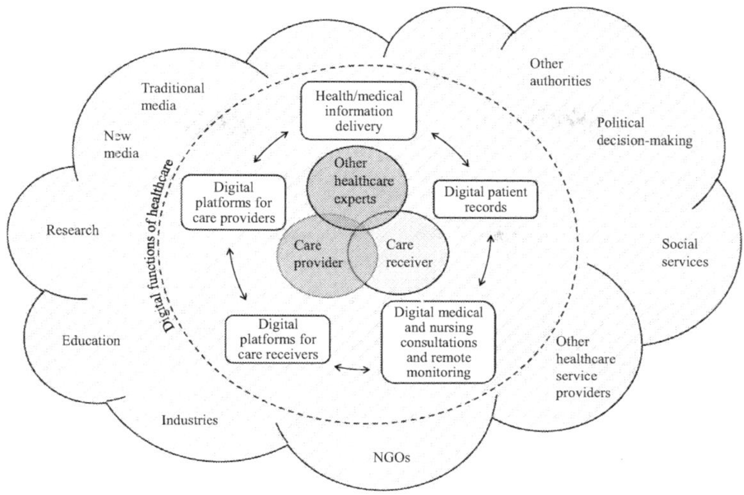

Figure 6.1 The communication environment of digital healthcare communication. Created by the authors.

for healthcare professionals will also change the division of labour, and, most likely, there will be ever more varied communicative tasks for care providers in the future. Furthermore, healthcare communication will also become more convoluted from a technological perspective, with more communication channels, platforms, and systems to take care of all this communication. Despite this increasing complexity in the communication format, the channel, platform, or system used for communication, and the communicators involved in the process, the core of healthcare communication always has been and always will be the interaction between the care provider and the care receiver.

References

Andreassen, H. K., Dyb, K., May, C. R., Pope, C. J., & Warth, L. L. (2018). Digitized patient–provider interaction: How does it matter? A qualitative meta-synthesis. *Social Science & Medicine*, *215*, 36–44. https://doi.org/10.1016/j.socscimed.2018.08.036

Bagger, C., Einarsson, A. M., Alvarez, V. A., Klausen, M., & Lomborg, S. (2023). Digital resignation and the datafied welfare state. *Big Data & Society*, *10*(2). https://doi.org/10.1177/20539517231206806

Buchert, U., Wrede, S., & Kouvonen, A. (2024). Persisting inequalities in the digitalized society: Migrant women facing coercive dimensions of everyday digitalization. *Communication & Society*, *27*(5), 935–950. https://doi.org/10.1080/1369118X.2023.2230265

Dickinson, R., Makowski, D., Van Marwijk, H., & Ford, E. (2025). Interventions for combating COVID-19 misinformation: A systematic realist review. *PLoS ONE*, *20*(4), e0321818. https://doi.org/10.1371/journal.pone.0321818

Do Nascimento, I. J. B., Pizarro, A. B., Almeida, J. M., Azzopardi-Muscat, N., Gonçalves, M. A., Björklund, M., & Novillo-Ortiz, D. (2022). Infodemics and health misinformation: A systematic review of reviews. *Bulletin of the World Health Organization*, *100*(9), 544–561. https://doi.org/10.2471/BLT.21.287654

Eden, D., & Bloor, J. (2010). Communication intelligence: Optimising healthcare communication in a digital age. *Journal of Communication in Healthcare*, *3*(2), 113–123. https://doi.org/10.1179/175380710X12813488575808

Eriksson-Backa, K., Ahmad, F., Huvila, I., Enwald, H., & Hirvonen, N. (2022). Everyday health information literacy and attitudes towards digital health services among Finnish older adults. In S. Kurbanoglu, S. Spiranec, Y. Ünal, J. Boustany, & D. Kos (Eds.), *Information literacy in a post-truth era – ECIL 2021* (pp. 314–325). Springer. https://doi.org/10.1007/978-3-030-99885-1_27

Heley, K., Chou, W.-Y. S., D'Angelo, H., Everson, N. S., Muro, A., Rohde, J. A., & Gaysynsky, A. (2025). Mitigating health and science misinformation: A scoping review of literature from 2017 to 2022. *Health Communication*, *40*(1), 79–89. https://doi.org/10.1080/10410236.2024.2332817

Hunter, R. F., De la Haye, K., Murray, J. M., Badham, J., Valente, T. W., Clarke, M., & Kee, F. (2019). Social network interventions for health behaviours and outcomes: A systematic review and meta-analysis. *PLoS Medicine*, *16*(9), e1002890. https://doi.org/10.1371/journal.pmed.1002890

Jæger, B. (2021). Digital citizenship – a review of the academic literature. *dms – der moderne staat – Zeitschrift für Public Policy, Recht und Management*, *14*(1), 24–42. https://doi.org/10.3224/dms.v14i1.09

Järvelin, K., Vakkari, P., Arvola, P., Baskaya, F., Järvelin, A., Kekäläinen, J., Keskustalo, H., Kumpulainen, S., Saastamoinen, M., Savolainen, R., & Sormunen, E. (2015). Task-based information interaction evaluation: The viewpoint of program theory. *ACM Transactions on Information Systems*, *33*(1), Article 3. https://doi.org/10.1145/2699660

Knöchelmann, A., Healy, K., Frese, T., Kantelhardt, E., Mikolajczyk, R., Meyer, G., Schildmann, J., Steckelberg, A., & Herke, M. (2024). User profiles in digitalized healthcare: Active, potential, and rejecting – a cross-sectional study using latent class analysis. *BMC Health Services Research*, *24*, 1083. https://doi.org/10.1186/s12913-024-11523-w

Marent, B., & Henwood, F. (2023). Digital health: A sociomaterial approach. *Sociology of Health & Illness*, *45*(1), 37–53. https://doi.org/10.1111/1467-9566.13538

Mort, M., Roberts, C., & Callén, B. (2013). Ageing with telecare: Care or coercion in austerity?. *Sociology of Health & Illness*, *35*(6), 799–812. https://doi.org/10.1111/j.1467-9566.2012.01530.x

Mossberger, K. (2008). Toward digital citizenship addressing inequality in the information age. In A. Chadwick & P. N. Howard (Eds.), *Routledge handbook of internet politics* (pp. 173–185). Routledge.

Mossberger, K., Tolbert, C. J., & McNeal, R. S. (2007). *Digital citizenship: The internet, society, and participation*. The MIT Press.

Neuberger, C., Bartsch, A., Fröhlich, R., Hanitzsch, T., Reinemann, C., & Schindler, J. (2023). The digital transformation of knowledge order: A model for the analysis of the epistemic crisis. *Annals of the International Communication Association*, *47*(2), 180–201. https://doi.org/10.1080/23808985.2023.2169950

Njenga, J. K. (2018). Digital literacy: The quest of an inclusive definition. *Reading & Writing*, *9*(1), a183. https://doi.org/10.4102/rw.v9i1.183

Rousaki, A., Zamani, E. D., Sbaffi, L., Hamblin, K., & Black, R. (2024). The digitalization of social care in England and implications for older, unpaid carers: Constructionist thematic analysis. *Journal of Medical Internet Research*, *26*, e60056. https://doi.org/10.2196/60056

Sendra, A., Torkkola, S., & Parviainen, J. (2024). AstraZeneca vaccine controversies in the media: Theorizing about the mediatization of ignorance in the context of the COVID-19 vaccination campaign. *Health Communication*, *39*(3), 541–551. https://doi.org/10.1080/10410236.2023.2171951

Stephens, M., & Mankee-Williams, A. (2021). The sickening truth of the digital divide: Digital health reforms and digital inequality. *Journal of Social Inclusion*, *12*(2), 57–66. https://journalofsocialinclusion.com/articles/10.36251/josi227

Talie Fenta, E., Bogale, E. K., & Anagaw, T. F. (2024). The role of social media on COVID-19 preventive behaviors worldwide, systematic review. *PLoS ONE*, *19*(7), e0306284. https://doi.org/10.1371/journal.pone.0306284

Torkkola, S. (2016). Multifaceted health communication. In V. Marinescu & B. Mitu (Eds.), *Health and the media: Essays on the effects of mass communication* (pp. 17–31). McFarland & Company, Inc.

Valkendorff, T., & Vanhatalo, U. (2025). Hospital personnel's experiences of using easy language in healthcare. A qualitative case study at a public hospital in Finland. *Journal of Communication in Healthcare*, *18*(1), 47–54. https://doi.org/10.1080/17538068.2024.2431771

WHO. (2021, December 6). *Health promotion glossary of terms 2021*. https://www.who.int/publications/i/item/9789240038349

Yildiz Durak, H., & Seferoğlu, S. S. (2020). Antecedents of social media usage status: Examination of predictiveness of digital literacy, academic performance, and fear of missing out variables. *Social Science Quarterly*, *101*(3), 1056–1074. https://doi.org/10.1111/ssqu.12790

Zhao, Y., & Wang, M. (2023). Digital sociology: Origin, development, and prospects from a global perspective. *The Journal of Chinese Sociology*, *10*, 19. https://doi.org/10.1186/s40711-023-00198-1

Index

Note: Page numbers in *italics* indicate a figure and page numbers in **bold** indicate a table on the corresponding page. Page numbers followed by "n" with numbers refer to notes.

Aamland, A. 29
Alinejad, D. 47
Alvarez-Galvez, J. 62
Alzghaibi, H. 7
Andreassen, H. K. 87
artificial intelligence (AI) 60–61, 70
Atanasoff, J. V. 5

Babaei, N. 58
Bagger, C. 86, 92
Barker, K. K. 61
being ill, experience of 38, 45; digitalizing 42–46, **42**; narratives to construct and make sense of 40–41; from perspective of patient 38–40, 46, 49, 70; from perspective of society 81–83, **85**, 86–89; understanding of 45
biomedical hegemony 23, 25
biomedicalization 79–80
The Birth of the Clinic (Foucault) 2–3, 59
Bloor, J. 30
Boorse, C. 27
Brennen, J. S. 5
Bury, M. 40–41

Cao, B. 45
Carel, H. 39
care provider 4, 6–7, 20, 24, 61, 66–70, 102; perspective of 9–10; *see also* care receiver
care receiver 2, 4, 6, 20, 24, 66–70, 102; conflict between care provider and 45–46; empowerment of 30; *see also* care provider
Chappell, Z. 27
Charon, R. 39
citizen 2, 4, 29, 79, 84, 89; digital health 92; individual behaviours of 47; self-determination rights of 68–69
Clarke, A. E. 79
client 2–4, 8, 41
communication: digital healthcare 30, 58–59, 105, *107*; organizational 6, 9, 18–20
communication and ill health 18–21, *20*, **21**, 106; biomedical model of 24; communicating 22–24, *23*; concept of 25; dimensions of 26, *26*, 29, 31n3; health and illness 24–29; patienthood in digital healthcare communication 30; *see also* ill health
communicative tasks, digitalization of 102–105, **103**
communicative constitution of organizations (CCO) 19
Conrad, P. 84
COVID-19 pandemic 2, 37, 43–44, 87–88, 90–92; AstraZeneca vaccine 90–92, 106; medical

dis- and misinformation 62–63; telemedicine 66
Cunningham-Burley, S. 84
customer 3–4, 24

Davin, S. 22
decision-making 61, 67–68
Deetz, S. 20
Dhawan, D. 48
digital gaze 10; *see also* medical gaze to digital gaze
digital health 7, 30, 58; interventions 5–6; literacy 8, 48, 100–101
digital health citizenship 85, 89–92, 101
digital healthcare services 30, 60–61, 80, 106; active users of 100; health/medical information and 91; as information retrieval systems 101–102; and virtual medical practices 65
digitalization 5–6, 10; *see also* digitization
digital literacy 68–69, 99–100; digital health literacy 8, 48, 100–101
digitization 5–6; *see also* digitalization
discrimination 27–28, 81
disease 1, 3, 26–27; classification scheme for 60; communicable 62–63; concept of 27; digitalization of 10, 66; naturalistic definition of 26–27; noncommunicable 62–63; perception of 59; regimes 41, 49–50; respatialization of 10, 66; retemporalization of 10–11, 66; signs of 10, 26–27, 29, 60, 70; supremacy of 41; triad of 10–11, 25, 31n3
disinformation 30; and misinformation 21, 46, 62–63, **103**, 104
Dutta, M. 9–10, 22–25
Dutton, W. H. 21

Eden, D. 30, 101
eHealth 7
electronic health records (EHRs) 6, 61
empowerment 11, 69, 89, 99, 106; rhetoric of 47; source for 30
Erikainen, S. 10, 41, 47
Eriksson, E. 49
experiential knowledge 38–39, 48, 51, 60; construction of 40, 46
expert knowledge 28, 38–39, 51
expertise 10, 26, *26*, 28, 39, 42–46, 49–51, 60; joint 69–70; of patients 51, 61

Farré, J. 43
Felt, U. 87
Foss, L. 58
Foucault, M. 7, 10, 58–59
Frank, A. W. 40–41
Fraser, S. 88

Gadamer, H.-G. 24, 59–60
Gonzalez-Polledo, E. 43, 45
Groleau, D. 83–84
Gybel Jensen, C. 8

health 4, 11n1, 23–24, 80; animal 4; authorities 106; campaigns 22; environmental 4; general theory of 25–26; human 4; literacy 100; and medical information 104–106; misinformation 62–63; state of 47
Health 2.0 7
health behaviour 22, 104; active 79–80; proper 80, 88–91, 106
healthcare communication 20; digitalization of 6–8; sub-fields of 9, 18–19, 31n1
healthcare experts 20; education of 104
healthcare organizations 49, 102, 106; collaborators of 30; health and medical information 104; and medical education providers 105; members of 20, 30; workload 105; *see also* healthcare professionals
healthcare professionals (HCPs) 45–46, 48, 50, 91; authority of

69, 105–106; communicative tasks for 106–107; education for 6, 10; expertise of 51; medical authorities and 62; reorientation of individual 102; superiority of 41; training of 63; trust in 49; *see also* healthcare organizations
healthcare services 4; digital opportunities for 105; provider/receiver of 20; provision of 6; users 20; virtual 66
health citizenship 9, 11, 29, 106; biomedicalization dimension of 83–84; concept of 83–85; digital 70, 81, 85–86, 89–91, 100; disconnected 86–87; distributed 88–89; enactment of 90–92; longevity of 90; performances of 80, 87; reconstruction of 80
health communication 18–19
health knowledge 104; co-construction of 50, 105; construction of 37, 39, 49
health professionalism 24, 30
health promotion 11, 29; and disease reduction 79; and illness care 22; personal responsibility for 70; principles of 81; self-care and 11, 84–85, 89, 91–92
Helén, I. 29, 83–84
Hilberg, E. 90
HIV criminalization 82–83
Ho, A. 60–61
Hofmann, B. 27, 31n3
Hogg, C. 3
Hoppe, T. 82–83
House of Babel (Jersild) 1, *2*, 8
Hut, L. 22
Hydén, L. 40–41

ignorance 61, 91
ill health 30, 23–25, 60, 70; biological manifestation of 57; "complete" absence of 4; multidimensionality of 29; plurality of 25
illness, digitalization of 37–38; chronic 40; consolidation of participatory patienthood 49–51; making sense of experience of being ill 40–41; experience of being ill 42–46, **42**; experience of being ill from the perspective of patient 38–40; narratives 40, 49; risks associated with 46–49
infomedicine 58
infrastructural factors 99–100
institutions 20, 24, 89–90, 92; and policymakers 81; social insurance 28
International Consortium of Investigative Journalists (ICIJ) 21
Internet 21, 30, 45–46, 61–62, 87, 99–100, 104
interpersonal communication 18–19, 20

Jæger, B. 101
Jauho, M. 29, 83–84
Jersild, P. C. 1, *2*, 8
journalism 18, 21

Khullar, D. 46
Kidd, I. J. 39
Klausen, M. 87, 89
Klawiter, M. 41
Knöchelmann, A. 100
knowledge: asymmetries 39; embodied 61; health 37, 49, 51, 80, 83, 104–105; medical 10, 28, 50, 60–61, 68, 105; personal 100; social 28; traditional dynamics of 61; uncomfortable 61
Kreiss, D. 5
Krishna, A. 48

Langdridge, D. 80, 87
Lee, S. 46
Lie, S. S. 92
Lupton, D. 9–10, 22, 43, 49

Magnussen, H. J. 39
Mankee-Williams, A. 99–100
Marshall, T. H. 29
Maslen, S. 43
mass communication 18–19, 20

May, C. 37
McCartney, G. 4
McPhee, R. D. 19–20
medical information 61, 100–101; and care services **69**; delivery 60–64, 102–103, 106; management of 60; sources of 63, 67
medicalization 9, 26, 28–29, 79
medical gaze to digital gaze 57–58; joint expertise 69–70, **69**; medical care 64–69, *64–65*; medical information delivery 60–64, **62**; modern medicine, birth of 58–60
medical knowledge 10, 50, 60–61, 68
medical practice 10, 39–40, 57, 60–61, 70; contemporary 41, 51; online 58; participatory 49
medicine 46; as art 10, 58, 105; evidence-based 43, 49, 60, 67; hegemonic status of 29; narrative 39–40; as science 10, 58, 105; social function of 79; value-free 23
Medicine 2.0 7, 58
Memenga, P. 48
m-health 7
Mills, C. 90
misinformation 48, 62, 91, 104; and disinformation 63, **69**
modern medicine 10, 27, 37, 51; birth of 58–60, 106
Mol, A. 66, 88
moral obligation 82–84, 90; of being well 11, 81, 87, 89, 91
Morris, W. *Artifact Panel* 31n2
Mumby, D. K. 20

Nordenfelt, L. 25–26
Nordtug, M. 91

obesity 81, 86
One Health 4–5
online communities 43; characteristics of 44; peer-led 42; potential of 44
organization 21; biomedical 79; bureaucratic 1; efficiency of 30; healthcare 11, 20, 30, 46, 49, 102, 104–106; patient 4, 81
organizational communication 19–20
Osborne, T. 59

Parsons, T. 27
partner 3–4
Parviainen, J. 61–62, **62**
patient 2–4, 27; concept of 50; –doctor relationships 44–45, 59–61; informed 69, 101, 105; satisfaction 68
patient-citizens 86–88, 91–92; ability of 91; objectivist-changer 88; semiotic-aesthetic 88; transformation of 86
patienthood 26–27; changes in 59; construction of 30, 59; digitalization of 105–107, *107*; exercise of 10, 42, 88; participatory 49–51; reconstruction of 59, 106; sociocultural understanding of 9, 11; visualization of 64–65, *64*
Payer, L. 57
Petersen, A. 86, 88
Petrakaki, D. 86, 89–90
Philosophy and Medicine (Gadamer) 24
Piera-Jiménez, J. 30
policymakers 81, 89–90, 92
Pols, J. 88
power: biomedicalization 79; medical knowledge and 28, 61, 69; relations 20, 23; relationship care provider vs. care receiver 4, 37, 41, 105; state, individual, market 11, 92
Putnam, L. L. 19

question-and-answer (Q&A) systems 61

Rayner, S. **62**
Raz, M. 62
Rembrandt, *The Anatomy Lesson of Dr. Nicolaes Tulp* 64, *65*

respatialization 7, 8, 10, 70, 87, 102
responsibility 79–80; for care 67, 106; personal 29, 70; professional 104; transferability of 30; virtual distribution of 88–89
retemporalization 7, 9, 10–11, 67, 102, 105
Ressler, P. K. 43
Rose, N. 58, 83–84
Rothenberg, K. 58
Rowe, F. 90

Sánchez-Carracedo, D. 81
SARS-CoV-2 infection 44
Schaller, S. 47
self-discipline 11, 89, 90, 92
Sendra, A. 43, 46, **62**
self-help digital mental health interventions (self-help DMHIs) 68
Sharf, B. F. 3–4
sickness, digitalization of 27–28, 31n3, 79–81; certification 82, 84; criminalization of 83; balanced digital health citizenship 91–92; experience of being ill from the perspective of society 81–83; health citizenship 83–85; health citizenship to digital health citizenship 85–89, **85**; relationship between empowerment and self-discipline 89–91
Sick Story: Research on Theory of Health Journalism and the Newspaper Hospital (Torkkola) 25
SNOMED CT 60
social media 21, 38, 39, 44–47, 100, 104
Song, M. 67
Sosnowy, C. 10, 43, 47
Stage, C. 42, 45
Stephens, M. 99–100
stigmatization 27–28, 47–48, 81
Street Jr, R. L. 3–4
Suarez-Lledo, V. 62

Tarr, J. 45
telecare 7
telemedicine 6, 58, 65–66, 105
therapeutic communication 18–19
Thompson, T. L. 48
Timmermans, S. 46
Torkkola, S. 23, *23*, 25, 31n3, **62**
Tretter, M. 90
Twaddle, A. 25, 27, 31n3

UNAIDS 82–83

Van Dijck, J. 47
Varey, S. 50
verbalization 27; of empathy 67
Virchow, R. 79
virtual healthcare 66; asynchronous telehealth 66–67; remote monitoring 66–67, 70, 105; synchronous telehealth 66
virtual medicine 10, 38, 58, 66–70

Wang, L. 45
well-being 44, 60, 80, 92
WHO 5, 11n1, 19, 63, 100

Zaug, P. 19–20

Made in the USA
Las Vegas, NV
19 September 2026

3fcb71d0-fabb-4d4c-9164-82dbe6333746R01